THE ULTIMATE ANTI-INFLAMMATORY DIET COOKBOOK

Savor Wellness, Transform Your Health, Indulge in 7-Day Meal Plans and Over 100 Recipes for a Blissful Journey to Vibrant Living

Dr. Kyla Brehm

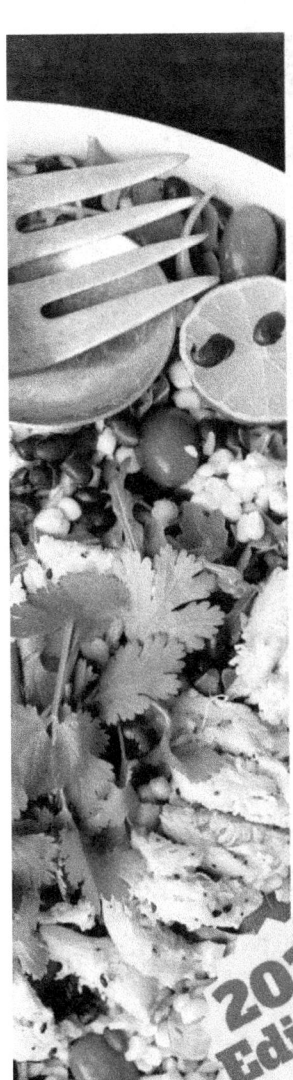
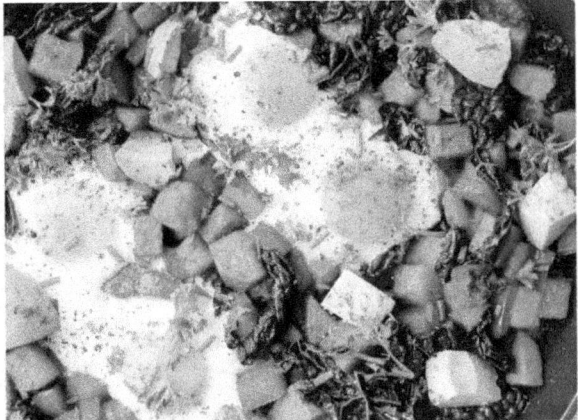

ANTI-INFLAMMATORY DIET
COOKBOOK

Savor Wellness, Transform Your Health!
Indulge, in 7-Day Meal Plans and Over 100
Recipes for a Blissful Journey to Vibrant Living

2024 Edition

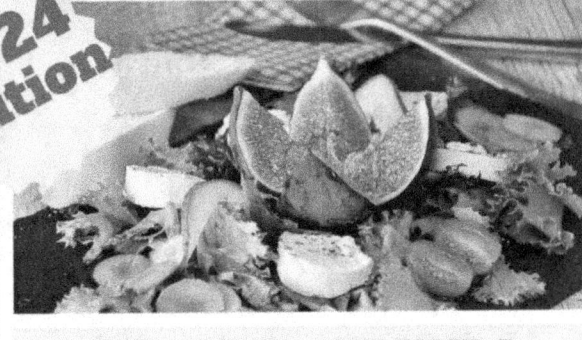

DR. KYLA BREHM

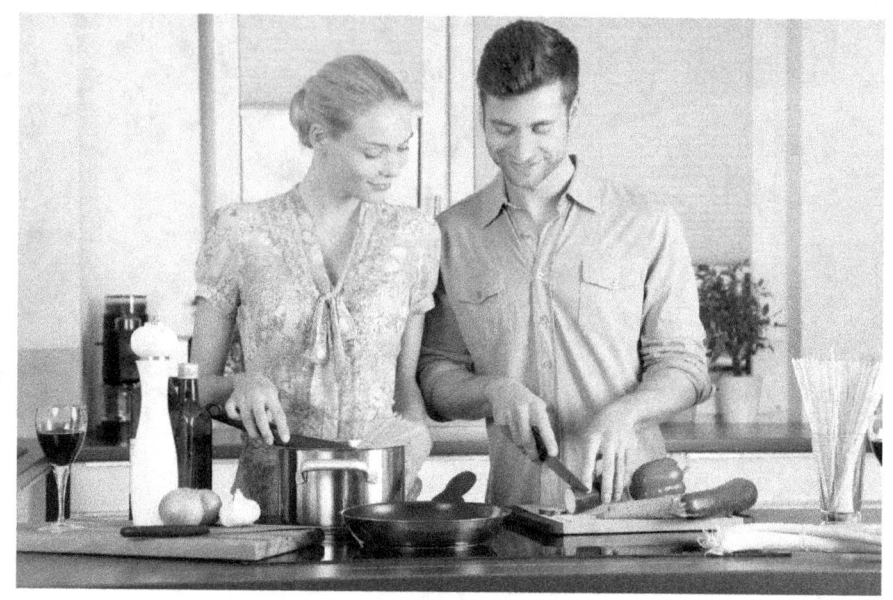

TABLE OF CONTENT

INTRODUCTION

Welcome to **"The Ultimate Anti-Inflammatory Diet Cookbook"** – a culinary journey crafted to redefine your relationship with food and transform your well-being. In a world inundated with fad diets, our cookbook stands out as a beacon of flavorful, sustainable health.

In today's fast-paced lives, where stress and processed foods dominate our choices, the need for a holistic approach to health has never been more crucial. This cookbook isn't just a collection of recipes; it's a roadmap to a life rich in vitality, where every meal becomes a moment of healing and delight.

Importance of Anti-Inflammatory Diets

Unlocking the secrets of inflammation is the cornerstone of this culinary exploration. We delve into the science behind inflammation, demystifying its impact on our health. This cookbook isn't a restrictive regimen; it's an invitation to embrace an anti-inflammatory lifestyle – a sustainable way to nourish your body, soothe ailments, and promote lasting wellness.

As you embark on this journey, envision your body as a canvas, and each recipe as a stroke of vibrant health. The significance of an anti-inflammatory diet extends beyond the plate; it's a transformative experience that influences your entire well-being.

Addressing Specific Health Goals

This cookbook is meticulously tailored for individuals who aren't just seeking recipes but are on a quest for a personalized wellness transformation. Whether you're managing chronic conditions, pursuing a healthier lifestyle, or simply seeking a more vibrant existence, "Anti-Inflammatory Diet" is designed with you in mind.

We understand the unique challenges faced by readers— from the time constraints of busy professionals to the varied dietary needs of families. Every recipe, every meal plan is curated to align with your specific health goals, making the journey towards wellness not just achievable but also indulgently delicious.

So, whether you're a health enthusiast, a busy professional, or someone navigating the complexities of dietary restrictions, this cookbook is your companion in a culinary adventure towards lasting well-being.

Welcome to a world where healing and flavor intertwine, where every bite is a step towards a healthier, happier you. Let the pages of "Anti-Inflammatory Diet" be the beginning of your savory journey to a life transformed through the joy of mindful and delicious living.

CHAPTER ONE

Understanding Inflammation

Embark on a fascinating journey into the very core of well-being with **"Anti-Inflammatory Diet."** In this chapter, we unravel the intricate science behind inflammation, demystifying its essence and exploring its profound impact on your health.

What is Inflammation?

At the heart of our exploration lies the understanding of inflammation, a natural response that, when balanced, safeguards our health. Dive into the science that underpins this biological phenomenon – from the cellular level to the intricate dance of molecules within your body. Discover the nuanced ways in which inflammation serves as both a guardian and a potential disruptor to your vitality.

As you navigate this scientific narrative, we make complex concepts accessible, ensuring you grasp the essentials. It's not just about understanding inflammation; it's about empowering you to make informed, health-conscious choices.

How Inflammation Affects Health

Transition from theory to application as we delve into the tangible effects of inflammation on your health. Uncover the intricate connections between inflammation and chronic conditions, from arthritis to cardiovascular issues. Learn how the foods you choose can either fuel inflammation or act as soothing agents, influencing the very fabric of your well-being.

This section is not a lecture but a guide – a bridge between knowledge and practical application. As you grasp the profound implications of inflammation, you'll gain insights that empower you to make conscious, health-supportive decisions in your culinary journey.

Case Studies: Real-Life Transformations

Witness the power of an anti-inflammatory lifestyle through the lens of real-life transformations. In this segment, we bring you stories of individuals who embraced the principles outlined in this cookbook and experienced tangible improvements in their health. These are not just success stories; they are testimonials to the transformative potential of mindful eating.

These case studies serve as beacons of inspiration, illustrating how individuals facing diverse health challenges navigated their unique paths to wellness. From increased energy levels to reduced inflammation-related discomfort, these stories showcase the tangible impact of incorporating anti-inflammatory practices into daily life.

As you turn the pages of **"Anti-Inflammatory Diet,"** remember that understanding inflammation isn't just about knowledge – it's a gateway to a more conscious and intentional approach to your health. Embrace the science, feel the effects, and let the real-life stories illuminate the path toward a vibrantly healthy you.

CHAPTER TWO

Simplifying the Anti-Inflammatory Diet

Welcome to the heart of **"Anti-Inflammatory Diet,"** where we demystify the intricate world of the anti-inflammatory diet. This chapter is your compass, guiding you through the essential elements that transform a collection of recipes into a comprehensive, accessible wellness strategy.

Demystifying Nutritional Concepts

We kick off by unraveling nutritional concepts, translating scientific jargon into practical wisdom. Whether you're a seasoned health enthusiast or just beginning your wellness journey, we ensure that the principles of the anti-inflammatory diet are presented in a manner that's both insightful and easily applicable.

No need for complicated charts or confusing terminology – we break it down to the essentials, empowering you to make informed choices that resonate with your individual health goals. In "Anti-Inflammatory Diet," simplicity doesn't compromise substance; it enhances it.

Grocery Shopping Guide: Essential Ingredients

Navigate the aisles with confidence as we provide you with a comprehensive grocery shopping guide. Discover the essential ingredients that form the foundation of an anti-inflammatory pantry. From vibrant fruits and vegetables to whole grains and lean proteins, our guide is a curated selection designed to simplify your shopping experience.

But it's not just about what to buy – we guide you on how to select the freshest produce, decipher food labels, and make choices that align with your health objectives. This section isn't just a list; it's your key to creating a kitchen stocked with ingredients that nourish both your body and your taste buds.

The essential ingredients for an anti-inflammatory diet, as outlined in "Anti-Inflammatory Diet," encompass a variety of food groups known for their anti-inflammatory properties. **Here's a brief overview:**

1. **Vibrant Fruits and Vegetables:** Rich in antioxidants, vitamins, and minerals, these form the colorful foundation of your diet. Berries, leafy

greens, cruciferous vegetables, and brightly colored fruits are key players.

2. **Whole Grains:** Opt for whole grains like quinoa, brown rice, oats, and barley. These provide complex carbohydrates, fiber, and essential nutrients without causing inflammation.

3. **Lean Proteins:** Choose lean protein sources such as fish (especially fatty fish like salmon), poultry, legumes, and tofu. These offer high-quality protein without excessive saturated fats.

4. **Healthy Fats:** Include sources of healthy fats, such as olive oil, avocados, and nuts. These fats have anti-inflammatory properties and contribute to overall heart health.

5. **Herbs and Spices:** Embrace the vibrant flavors and anti-inflammatory benefits of herbs and spices. Turmeric, ginger, garlic, and cinnamon are notable additions known for their health-promoting properties.

6. **Nuts and Seeds:** Almonds, walnuts, chia seeds, and flaxseeds are excellent sources of healthy fats, omega-3 fatty acids, and antioxidants.

7. **Probiotic-Rich Foods:** Incorporate fermented foods like yogurt, kefir, and sauerkraut. These support gut health, influencing overall inflammation levels in the body.

8. **Colorful Herbs and Teas:** Explore the benefits of herbs like chamomile and green tea, known for their anti-inflammatory and antioxidant properties.

Remember, the key is to create a well-rounded and diverse diet that incorporates a variety of these essential ingredients. "Anti-Inflammatory Diet" provides a detailed guide, ensuring you have the right components to embark on a delicious and anti-inflammatory culinary journey.

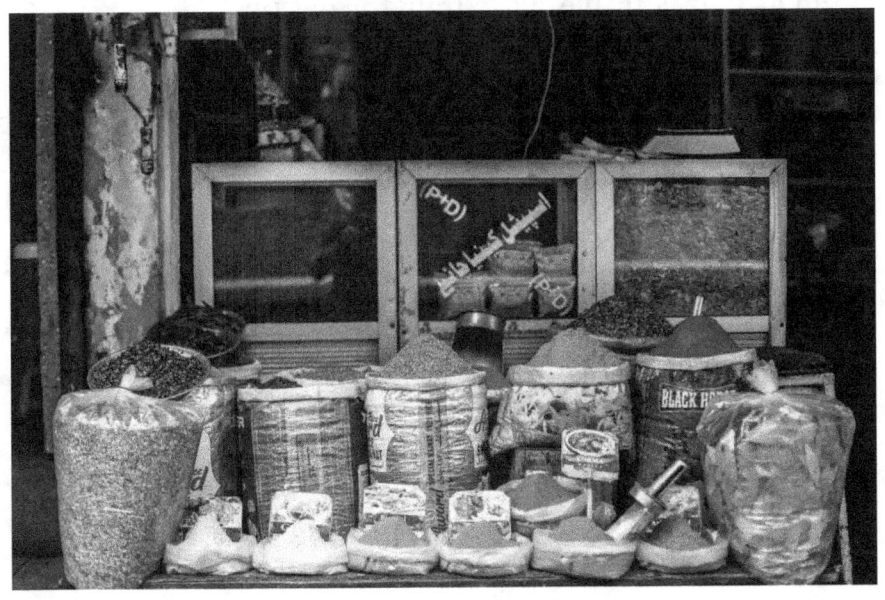

Kitchen Essentials for a Healing Culinary Journey

Your kitchen is not just a place to cook; it's a sanctuary of healing. We guide you through the essential tools and equipment that transform your culinary space into a therapeutic haven. From efficient chopping techniques to mastering the art of nutrient retention through cooking methods, this section ensures that your kitchen becomes an ally in your wellness transformation.

Explore the synergy between the right tools and the right ingredients, creating a space where the act of preparing meals becomes a joyful and healthful ritual. In "Anti-Inflammatory Diet," we prioritize not just what goes on your plate but the environment in which it is crafted.

In "Anti-Inflammatory Diet," the kitchen essentials refer to the tools and equipment that enhance your culinary experience, making it both practical and enjoyable. **Here are some kitchen essentials highlighted in the book:**

1. **Sharp Knives:** Invest in high-quality, sharp knives for efficient and precise chopping, slicing, and dicing.

2. **Cutting Boards:** Use cutting boards made from materials like bamboo or high-density polyethylene to provide a hygienic and sturdy surface.

3. **Cookware:** Essential pots and pans made from materials like stainless steel or cast iron, ensuring even heat distribution and durability.

4. **Utensils:** A set of cooking utensils, including spatulas, ladles, and tongs, designed for various cooking tasks.

5. **Blender or Food Processor:** For smoothies, sauces, and purees, a reliable blender or food processor can be a versatile addition to your kitchen.

6. **Measuring Tools:** Accurate measuring cups and spoons for precise ingredient quantities, especially crucial in baking.

7. **Cutting Techniques Guide:** Tips and techniques for efficient and safe chopping, mincing, and other cutting methods.

8. **Cooking Methods Guide:** Insight into cooking methods that help retain nutrients in your ingredients, ensuring a healthful approach to meal preparation.

9. **Storage Containers:** Containers for storing prepped ingredients or leftovers, promoting an organized and efficient kitchen.

10. **Cooking Techniques for Nutrient Retention:** Guidance on methods like steaming, sautéing, or roasting to preserve the nutritional value of your foods.

By incorporating these kitchen essentials, "Anti-Inflammatory Diet" aims to transform your kitchen into a space that supports your health and well-being, making the act of preparing meals a joyful and nourishing

experience.

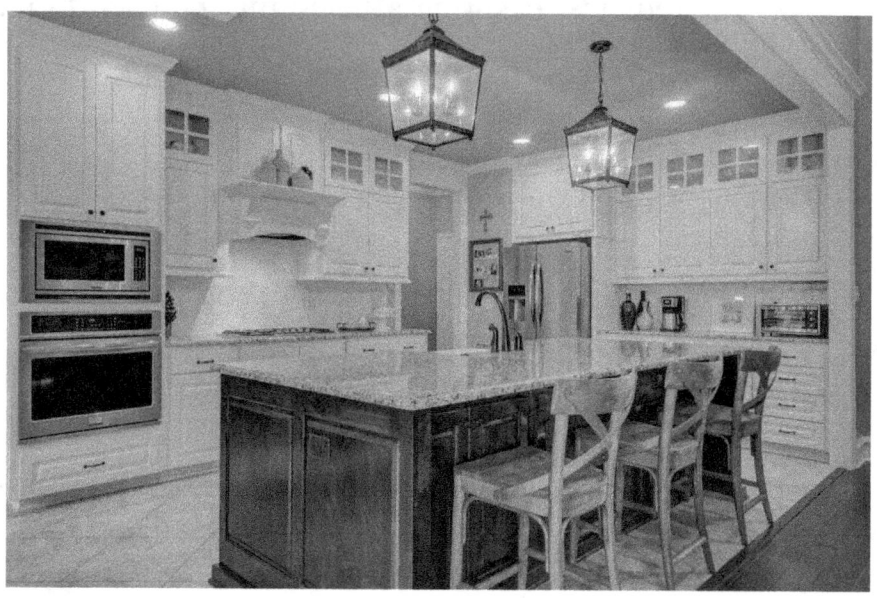

CHAPTER THREE

7-Day Wellness Transformation

Embark on a transformative journey with "Anti-Inflammatory Diet" as we guide you through a week-long immersion into the healing wonders of an anti-inflammatory diet. In this chapter, we present meticulously crafted day-wise meal plans, accompanied by nutritional insights and invaluable tips to ensure your success on this vibrant path to wellness.

Day-wise Meal Plans: Breakfast, Lunch, Dinner, Snacks

Picture waking up to a breakfast that not only delights your taste buds but sets a positive tone for the day. "Anti-Inflammatory Diet" brings you seven days of thoughtfully curated meal plans, each comprising nourishing breakfasts, invigorating lunches, satisfying dinners, and guilt-free snacks. From energizing smoothie bowls to savory one-pan dinners, every meal is a celebration of flavor and well-being.

No need to worry about monotonous or complicated recipes – we've carefully designed these meal plans to be not only delicious but also feasible for your daily routine. Whether you're a culinary enthusiast or someone with a busy schedule, these plans ensure that every bite is a step towards your wellness goals.

7-days Meal Plan

Below is a sample 7-day meal plan from **"Anti-Inflammatory Diet Cookbook,"** designed to showcase a variety of delicious and anti-inflammatory recipes. Please note that individual dietary needs may vary, and it's always a good idea to consult with a healthcare professional or nutritionist for personalized advice.

Day 1:

- **Breakfast:** Berry and Spinach Smoothie Bowl with Almond Butter

- **Lunch:** Quinoa Salad with Mixed Vegetables and Grilled Chicken

- **Dinner:** Baked Salmon with Lemon and Herbs, Roasted Sweet Potatoes, and Steamed Broccoli

- **Snack:** Greek Yogurt Parfait with Berries and a Sprinkle of Chia Seeds

Day 2:

- **Breakfast:** Avocado and Tomato Toast on Whole Grain Bread

- **Lunch:** Lentil and Vegetable Soup with a Side of Mixed Greens

- **Dinner:** Stir-Fried Tofu with Vegetables and Brown Rice

- **Snack:** Sliced Cucumber with Hummus

Day 3:

- **Breakfast:** Overnight Oats with Mixed Berries and a Drizzle of Honey

- **Lunch:** Quinoa Stuffed Bell Peppers with Ground Turkey

- **Dinner:** Grilled Shrimp Skewers, Quinoa Pilaf, and Roasted Asparagus

- **Snack:** Apple Slices with Almond Butter

Day 4:

- **Breakfast:** Spinach and Feta Omelette with Whole Grain Toast

- **Lunch:** Chickpea and Vegetable Curry with Brown Basmati Rice

- **Dinner:** Baked Chicken Breast with Turmeric, Roasted Brussels Sprouts, and Cauliflower Mash

- **Snack:** Trail Mix with Nuts and Dried Fruit

Day 5:

- **Breakfast:** Banana Walnut Pancakes (Whole Grain or Gluten-Free)

- **Lunch:** Quinoa and Black Bean Bowl with Avocado and Lime Dressing

- **Dinner:** Cod Fish Tacos with Cabbage Slaw and Mango Salsa

- **Snack:** Cottage Cheese with Pineapple Chunks

Day 6:

- **Breakfast:** Chia Seed Pudding with Mango and Coconut

- **Lunch:** Mediterranean Salad with Grilled Chicken, Olives, and Feta

- **Dinner:** Eggplant and Chickpea Stew with Quinoa

- **Snack:** Cherry Tomatoes with Mozzarella Cheese

Day 7:

- **Breakfast:** Green Tea Smoothie with Kale, Pineapple, and Ginger

- **Lunch:** Turkey and Vegetable Wrap with Whole Grain Tortilla

- **Dinner:** Baked Halibut with Herb Crust, Roasted Sweet Potato Wedges, and Green Beans

- **Snack:** Mixed Berries and a Handful of Almonds

Feel free to adapt this meal plan based on your preferences and dietary requirements. Each day is crafted to provide a balance of nutrients and delicious flavors, contributing to your overall well-being.

Nutritional Insights for Each Day

Beyond the delightful recipes, each day comes with nutritional insights tailored to enhance your understanding of the benefits behind the chosen ingredients. Explore the synergy of nutrients, discover the anti-inflammatory properties of key components, and gain insights into how each meal contributes to your overall well-being.

"Anti-Inflammatory Diet" is not just a cookbook; it's a holistic guide that empowers you to make informed choices about what goes on your plate. We break down the nutritional content in a way that's accessible and engaging, fostering a deeper connection between your food and your health.

Tips for Success: Staying on Track Throughout the Week

Embarking on a wellness transformation may seem daunting, but fear not – we've compiled a wealth of tips to ensure your success throughout the week. From practical meal-prep strategies to mindful eating practices, these tips are your companions in navigating the intricacies of an anti-inflammatory lifestyle.

"Anti-Inflammatory Diet" is not about rigid rules but flexible guidelines that adapt to your lifestyle. Whether you're at home or on the go, these tips provide the support you need to stay on track. Embrace the journey, savor each meal, and let these tips be the guiding light towards a week of transformative wellness.

As you immerse yourself in Chapter 3, envision a week where each day unfolds with purpose and flavor. Let "Anti-Inflammatory Diet" be your companion in this 7-day wellness transformation, where every meal is a delicious step towards a healthier, more vibrant you.

CHAPTER FOUR

Culinary Medicine in Action

Welcome to the heart of "Anti-Inflammatory Diet," where we dive deep into the realm of culinary medicine, demonstrating how your kitchen can become a powerhouse of healing. This chapter is an ode to the art of crafting flavorful and therapeutic dishes, utilizing key healing ingredients and culinary techniques that maximize nutrient retention.

Highlighting Key Healing Ingredients

In this culinary journey, we shine a spotlight on ingredients celebrated not just for their flavors but for their profound healing properties. From the vibrant hues of turmeric, known for its anti-inflammatory benefits, to the robust antioxidants found in berries, each ingredient is carefully chosen for its potential to nourish and support your well-being.

"Anti-Inflammatory Diet" isn't just a collection of recipes; it's a guide to curating your pantry with ingredients that double as culinary medicine. Discover how the synergy of these elements can elevate your dishes, turning every meal into a delightful step towards health.

In "Anti-Inflammatory Diet," the key healing ingredients are carefully selected for their nutritional properties and potential health benefits. Here's a glimpse into some of the featured ingredients that play a crucial role in enhancing the therapeutic aspects of the recipes:

1. **Turmeric:** Known for its active compound curcumin, turmeric possesses powerful anti-inflammatory and antioxidant properties.

2. **Berries (e.g., Blueberries, Strawberries):** Packed with antioxidants, vitamins, and fiber, berries contribute to overall well-being and support immune health.

3. **Ginger:** Renowned for its anti-inflammatory and digestive properties, ginger adds a zing of flavor and therapeutic benefits to dishes.

4. **Leafy Greens (e.g., Spinach, Kale):** Rich in vitamins, minerals, and antioxidants, leafy greens are nutritional powerhouses that support various aspects of health.

5. **Salmon:** A fatty fish rich in omega-3 fatty acids, promoting heart health and contributing to anti-inflammatory effects.

6. **Quinoa:** A versatile whole grain, quinoa is a complete protein source and provides essential nutrients like fiber and minerals.

7. **Nuts and Seeds (e.g., Almonds, Chia Seeds):** Packed with healthy fats, fiber, and various nutrients, nuts and seeds contribute to a well-rounded diet.

8. **Garlic:** Beyond its flavorful addition to dishes, garlic has immune-boosting and anti-inflammatory properties.

9. **Olive Oil:** A source of healthy monounsaturated fats and antioxidants, olive oil is a staple in promoting heart health.

10. **Cauliflower:** High in fiber and rich in vitamins, cauliflower is a versatile vegetable that adds nutritional value to various recipes.

These key healing ingredients are strategically integrated into the recipes in "Anti-Inflammatory Diet," aiming not just to enhance flavor but also to provide a culinary medicine approach to well-being. Each ingredient is chosen for its potential to contribute to a balanced and healthful diet, supporting the overall goals of the anti-inflammatory journey outlined in the cookbook.

Cooking Techniques for Maximum Nutrient Retention

Master the art of cooking for health with techniques that go beyond flavor – they prioritize the preservation of essential nutrients. Whether it's the gentle steam that keeps vegetables vibrant or the precise grilling that locks in the juiciness of lean proteins, these techniques ensure that your dishes are not just delicious but also brimming with nutritional value.

This section isn't a mere list of instructions; it's a culinary education that empowers you to make conscious choices in the kitchen. Learn how to preserve the goodness in every bite, making your meals not only a feast for your taste buds but a nourishing ritual for your body.

Crafting Flavorful and Therapeutic Dishes

"Anti-Inflammatory Diet" is a testament to the idea that therapeutic dishes can be irresistibly flavorful. Explore recipes that go beyond mere sustenance, infusing your meals with a symphony of tastes and aromas. From aromatic herb-infused oils to spice blends that awaken the senses, each dish is a celebration of both culinary artistry and healing intention.

As you embark on crafting these dishes, embrace the joy of creating meals that not only nurture your body but also indulge your palate. Let your kitchen be a canvas where the brushstrokes of healing ingredients and mindful cooking techniques come together to create a masterpiece of flavor and well-being.

Chapter 4 invites you to experience the transformative power of culinary medicine, where your kitchen becomes not just a space for cooking but a sanctuary for health and joy. Let "Anti-Inflammatory Diet" be your guide to the delicious intersection of culinary art and medicinal nourishment.

CHAPTER FIVE

Recipe Showcase

Breakfast Delights: Start Your Day Right

Here are 10 breakfast recipes from "Anti-Inflammatory Diet," each crafted to start your day with delicious and nutritious delights:

1. Golden Turmeric Smoothie Bowl

Description: Start your day with a burst of sunshine! This golden turmeric smoothie bowl is not only visually appealing but also loaded with anti-inflammatory benefits, thanks to the star ingredient – turmeric.

Serving Size: 1 bowl

Prep Time: 10 minutes

Cooking Time: 0 minutes

Ingredients:

- 1 frozen banana

- 1/2 cup pineapple chunks

- 1/2 teaspoon turmeric powder

- 1/2 cup Greek yogurt

- 1/4 cup almond milk

- Toppings: Fresh berries, granola, chia seeds

Instructions:

1. Blend frozen banana, pineapple, turmeric powder, Greek yogurt, and almond milk until smooth.

2. Pour into a bowl and top with fresh berries, granola, and a sprinkle of chia seeds.

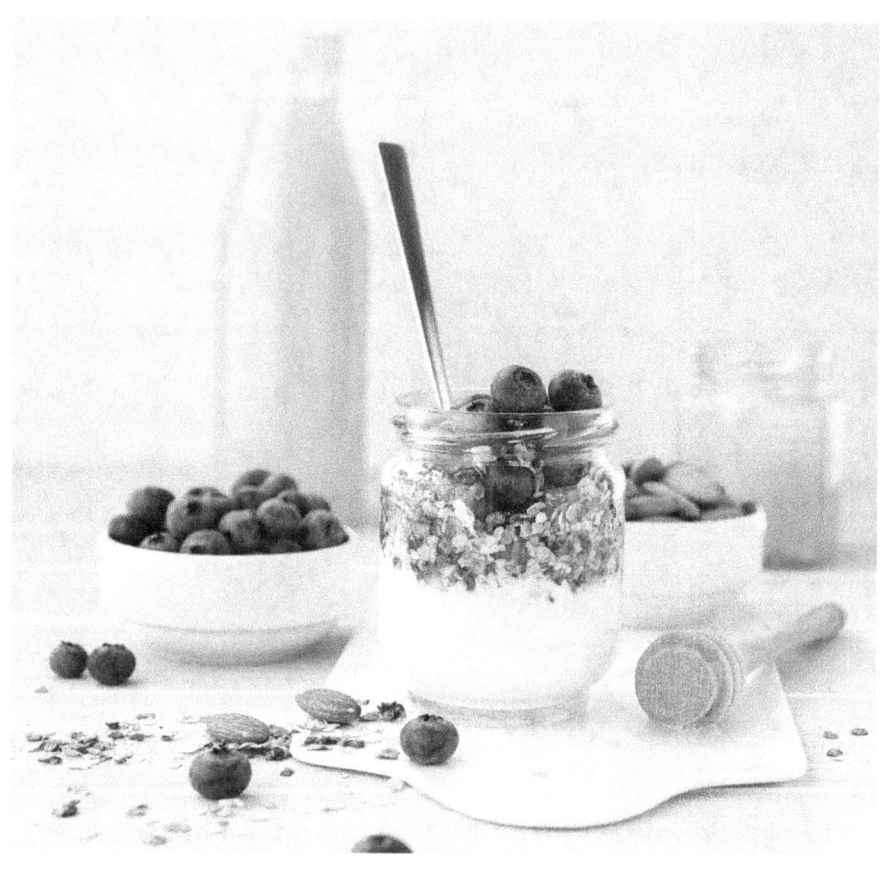

2. Spinach and Feta Omelette with Tomato Basil Salsa

Description: Elevate your breakfast routine with this nutrient-packed omelette. The combination of spinach, feta, and a vibrant tomato basil salsa creates a flavor explosion on your plate.

Serving Size: 1 omelette

Prep Time: 5 minutes

Cooking Time: 10 minutes

Ingredients:

- 2 large eggs

- Handful of fresh spinach, chopped

- 2 tablespoons feta cheese, crumbled

- 1 medium tomato, diced

- Fresh basil leaves, chopped

- Salt and pepper to taste

Instructions:

1. Whisk eggs and season with salt and pepper.

2. In a non-stick pan, sauté chopped spinach until wilted.

3. Pour whisked eggs over spinach, add feta, and cook until set.

4. In a bowl, mix diced tomato and basil for the salsa.

5. Fold the omelette, top with tomato basil salsa, and serve.

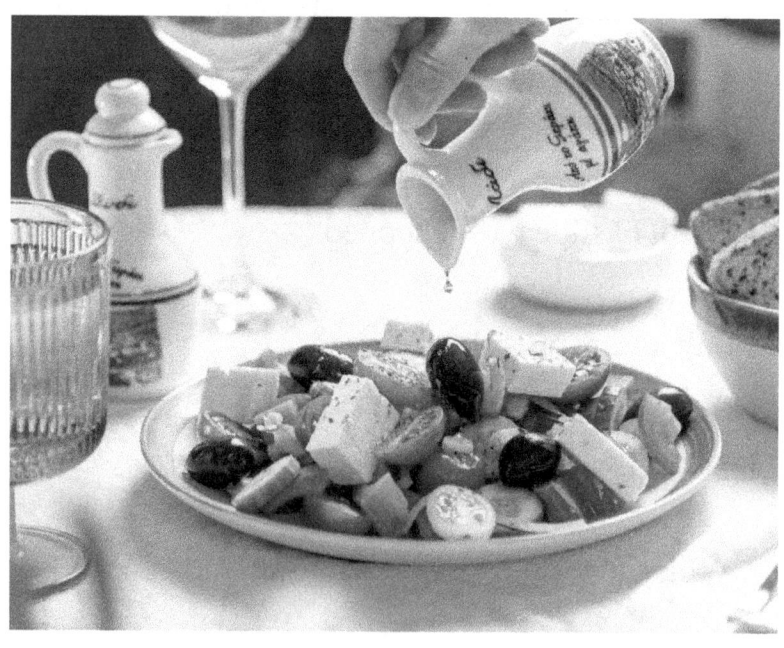

3. Berry Almond Overnight Oats

Description: Prepare your breakfast the night before with these delicious and satisfying overnight oats. The combination of berries and almonds provides a delightful crunch and natural sweetness.

Serving Size: 1 jar

Prep Time: 5 minutes (plus overnight soaking)

Cooking Time: 0 minutes

Ingredients:

- 1/2 cup rolled oats

- 1/2 cup almond milk

- 1/4 cup mixed berries (strawberries, blueberries, raspberries)

- 1 tablespoon almond butter

- 1 teaspoon honey

- Sliced almonds for topping

Instructions:

1. In a jar, combine oats, almond milk, berries, almond butter, and honey.

2. Stir well, cover, and refrigerate overnight.

3. In the morning, give it a good stir, top with sliced almonds, and enjoy.

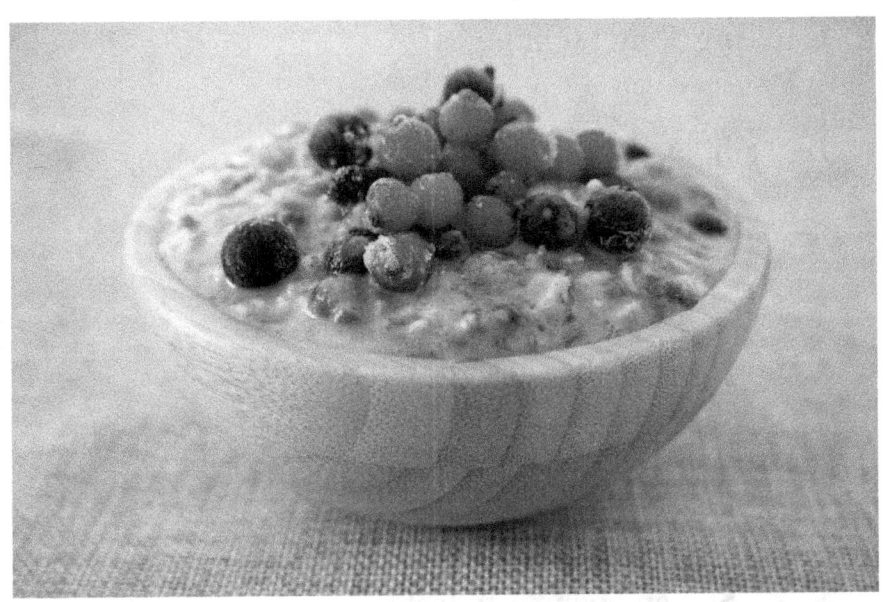

4. Avocado and Tomato Toast on Whole Grain Bread

Description: This avocado and tomato toast is a celebration of simplicity and freshness. Creamy avocado meets juicy tomatoes on wholesome whole grain bread for a delightful and nutritious breakfast.

Serving Size: 1 toast

Prep Time: 5 minutes

Cooking Time: 0 minutes

Ingredients:

- 1 slice whole grain bread, toasted

- 1/2 ripe avocado, mashed

- 1 medium tomato, sliced

- Salt and pepper to taste

- Optional: Red pepper flakes for a kick

Instructions:

1. Toast the whole grain bread to your liking.

2. Spread mashed avocado evenly on the toast.

3. Arrange tomato slices on top, sprinkle with salt, pepper, and red pepper flakes if desired.

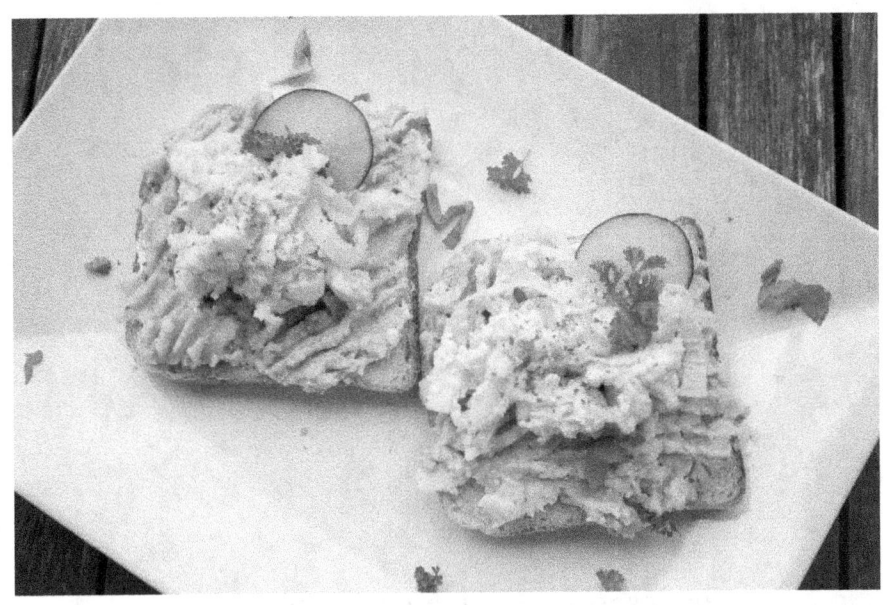

5. Chia Seed Pudding with Mango and Coconut

Description: Indulge in a tropical escape with this chia seed pudding featuring sweet mango and coconut. It's not only a treat for your taste buds but also a nutritious powerhouse.

Serving Size: 1 jar

Prep Time: 5 minutes (plus chilling time)

Cooking Time: 0 minutes

Ingredients:

- 2 tablespoons chia seeds

- 1/2 cup coconut milk

- 1/2 cup diced mango

- 1 tablespoon shredded coconut

- Drizzle of honey for sweetness

Instructions:

1. In a jar, combine chia seeds and coconut milk. Stir well and refrigerate for a few hours or overnight.

2. Layer chia pudding with diced mango and shredded coconut.

3. Drizzle honey on top and enjoy this tropical delight.

6. Banana Walnut Pancakes (Whole Grain or Gluten-Free)

Description: These banana walnut pancakes are a wholesome and comforting breakfast option. Whether you opt for whole grain or gluten-free, they promise a delightful start to your day.

Serving Size: 2 pancakes

Prep Time: 10 minutes

Cooking Time: 10 minutes

Ingredients:

- 1 ripe banana, mashed

- 2 eggs

- 1/2 cup whole grain flour or gluten-free flour

- 1/2 teaspoon baking powder

- Handful of chopped walnuts

- Maple syrup for drizzling

Instructions:

1. In a bowl, mix mashed banana and eggs until well combined.

2. Add flour and baking powder, stirring until smooth.

3. Fold in chopped walnuts.

4. Heat a griddle or non-stick pan, pour batter to make pancakes, and cook until golden brown on both sides.

5. Serve with a drizzle of maple syrup.

7. Blueberry Almond Smoothie

Description: Kickstart your day with a refreshing blueberry almond smoothie. Packed with antioxidants and protein, this smoothie is a delicious way to fuel your morning.

Serving Size: 1 glass

Prep Time: 5 minutes

Cooking Time: 0 minutes

Ingredients:

- 1/2 cup blueberries (fresh or frozen)

- 1/2 banana

- 1/4 cup plain Greek yogurt

- 1 tablespoon almond butter

- 1/2 cup almond milk

- Ice cubes (optional)

Instructions:

1. Blend blueberries, banana, Greek yogurt, almond butter, and almond milk until smooth.

2. Add ice cubes if desired and blend again.

3. Pour into a glass and savor the goodness.

8. Egg and Veggie Breakfast Wrap

Description: This egg and veggie breakfast wrap is a perfect on-the-go option, combining protein-packed eggs with a medley of colorful vegetables for a wholesome start to your day.

Serving Size: 1 wrap

Prep Time: 10 minutes

Cooking Time: 5 minutes

Ingredients:

- 2 large eggs, beaten

- 1 whole-grain or gluten-free wrap

- 1/4 cup diced bell peppers (mixed colors)

- 1/4 cup cherry tomatoes, halved

- Handful of spinach leaves

- Salt and pepper to taste

- Optional: Salsa or hot sauce for extra flavor

Instructions:

1. In a pan, sauté bell peppers until slightly softened.

2. Add cherry tomatoes and spinach, cooking until spinach wilts.

3. Push veggies to one side of the pan and pour beaten eggs into the other side.

4. Scramble eggs until cooked through, then mix with veggies.

5. Season with salt and pepper, and fill the wrap with the egg and veggie mixture.

6. Optional: Add salsa or hot sauce for an extra kick.

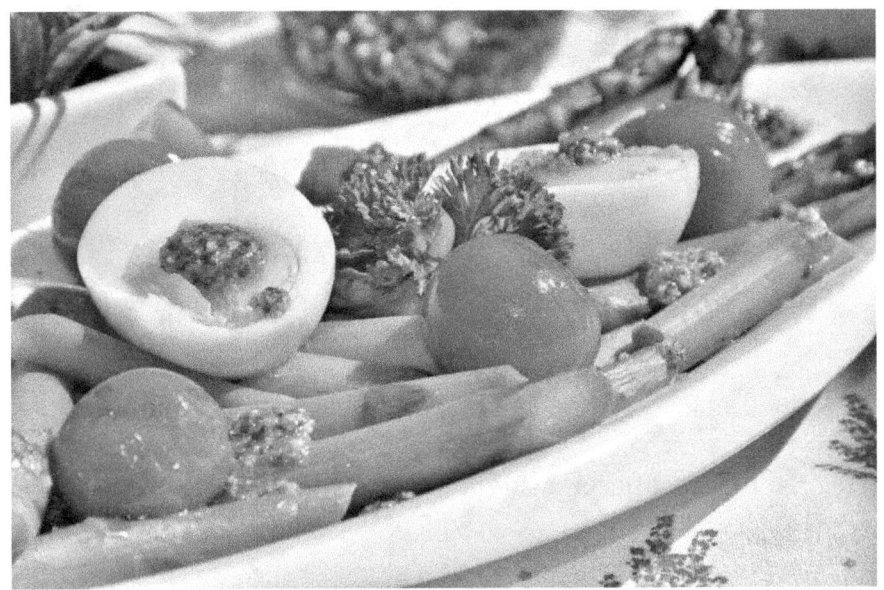

9. Peanut Butter and Banana Toast with Cinnamon

Description: Satisfy your taste buds with this classic combination of peanut butter and banana on whole grain toast. A sprinkle of cinnamon adds warmth and an extra layer of flavor.

Serving Size: 1 toast

Prep Time: 5 minutes

Cooking Time: 0 minutes

Ingredients:

- 1 slice whole grain bread, toasted

- 1 tablespoon peanut butter

- 1/2 banana, sliced

- Pinch of ground cinnamon

Instructions:

1. Toast the whole grain bread.

2. Spread peanut butter evenly on the toast.

3. Arrange banana slices on top and sprinkle with ground cinnamon.

10. Coconut Mango Parfait

Description: Indulge in a tropical paradise with this coconut mango parfait. Layers of creamy Greek yogurt, sweet mango, and crunchy granola create a delightful symphony of textures and flavors.

Serving Size: 1 parfait

Prep Time: 10 minutes

Cooking Time: 0 minutes

Ingredients:

- 1/2 cup Greek yogurt

- 1/2 cup diced mango

- 2 tablespoons shredded coconut

- 1/4 cup granola

- Drizzle of honey for sweetness

Instructions:

1. In a glass or bowl, layer Greek yogurt, diced mango, shredded coconut, and granola.

2. Repeat the layers until you reach the top.

3. Drizzle honey on top and enjoy this tropical parfait.

These breakfast recipes from "Anti-Inflammatory Diet" are designed to provide a mix of flavors, textures, and nutrients, ensuring a delightful and nutritious start to your day. Feel free to adapt them based on your preferences and dietary needs.

Lunchtime Favorites: Energize Your Afternoons

Here are 10 lunch recipes from "Anti-Inflammatory Diet" that are sure to energize your afternoons with a mix of vibrant flavors and wholesome ingredients:

1. Mediterranean Chickpea Salad

Description: Transport yourself to the shores of the Mediterranean with this refreshing chickpea salad. Bursting with colorful vegetables, feta cheese, and a zesty dressing, it's a satisfying and nutritious lunch option.

Serving Size: 2 servings

Prep Time: 15 minutes

Cooking Time: 0 minutes

Ingredients:

- 1 can (15 oz) chickpeas, drained and rinsed

- 1 cup cherry tomatoes, halved

- 1 cucumber, diced

- 1/2 red onion, finely chopped

- 1/2 cup Kalamata olives, sliced

- 1/2 cup feta cheese, crumbled

- 2 tablespoons extra virgin olive oil

- 1 tablespoon red wine vinegar

- Salt and pepper to taste

- Fresh oregano for garnish

Instructions:

1. In a large bowl, combine chickpeas, cherry tomatoes, cucumber, red onion, olives, and feta cheese.

2. In a small bowl, whisk together olive oil, red wine vinegar, salt, and pepper.

3. Pour the dressing over the salad and toss gently to combine.

4. Garnish with fresh oregano and serve.

2. Teriyaki Salmon Bowl with Quinoa

Description: Elevate your lunch with this teriyaki salmon bowl featuring succulent grilled salmon, vibrant vegetables, and nutrient-packed quinoa. A harmonious blend of flavors and textures in every bite.

Serving Size: 2 servings

Prep Time: 20 minutes

Cooking Time: 15 minutes

Ingredients:

- 2 salmon fillets

- 1/4 cup teriyaki sauce

- 1 cup quinoa, cooked

- 1 cup broccoli florets, steamed

- 1 carrot, julienned

- 1/2 red bell pepper, sliced

- 1 tablespoon sesame seeds

- Green onions for garnish

Instructions:

1. Marinate salmon fillets in teriyaki sauce for 10 minutes.

2. Grill salmon until cooked through, brushing with additional teriyaki sauce.

3. In bowls, assemble quinoa, steamed broccoli, julienned carrot, and sliced bell pepper.

4. Top with grilled salmon, sprinkle sesame seeds, and garnish with green onions.

3. Caprese Grilled Chicken Salad

Description: Experience the classic Caprese salad in a satisfying grilled chicken form. Fresh tomatoes, mozzarella, and basil combine with grilled chicken for a light yet filling lunch option.

Serving Size: 2 servings

Prep Time: 15 minutes

Cooking Time: 15 minutes

Ingredients:

- 2 boneless, skinless chicken breasts

- 1 tablespoon olive oil

- Salt and pepper to taste

- 2 large tomatoes, sliced

- 1 cup fresh mozzarella balls

- Fresh basil leaves

- Balsamic glaze for drizzling

Instructions:

1. Season chicken breasts with salt and pepper, then grill until cooked.

2. Slice grilled chicken into strips.

3. On a plate, arrange sliced tomatoes, mozzarella balls, and grilled chicken.

4. Garnish with fresh basil leaves and drizzle with balsamic glaze.

4. Vegetarian Quinoa-Stuffed Bell Peppers

Description: Elevate your lunch with these colorful vegetarian quinoa-stuffed bell peppers. Packed with a flavorful quinoa and vegetable filling, they are a wholesome and satisfying meal.

Serving Size: 4 servings

Prep Time: 20 minutes

Cooking Time: 30 minutes

Ingredients:

- 4 bell peppers, halved and seeds removed

- 1 cup quinoa, cooked

- 1 can (15 oz) black beans, drained and rinsed

- 1 cup corn kernels (fresh or frozen)

- 1 cup cherry tomatoes, halved

- 1/2 cup red onion, finely chopped

- 1 cup shredded cheddar cheese

- 1 teaspoon cumin

- 1 teaspoon chili powder

- Salt and pepper to taste

- Fresh cilantro for garnish

Instructions:

1. Preheat the oven to 375°F (190°C).

2. In a large bowl, mix cooked quinoa, black beans, corn, cherry tomatoes, red onion, shredded cheddar, cumin, chili powder, salt, and pepper.

3. Stuff bell pepper halves with the quinoa mixture.

4. Bake for 25-30 minutes or until peppers are tender.

5. Garnish with fresh cilantro and serve.

5. Asian-Inspired Beef and Broccoli Stir-Fry

Description: Take a trip to Asia with this flavorful beef and broccoli stir-fry. Tender slices of beef, crisp broccoli, and a savory sauce come together in a quick and satisfying lunch.

Serving Size: 2 servings

Prep Time: 15 minutes

Cooking Time: 15 minutes

Ingredients:

- 1/2 lb flank steak, thinly sliced

- 2 cups broccoli florets

- 1 red bell pepper, thinly sliced

- 2 tablespoons soy sauce

- 1 tablespoon oyster sauce

- 1 tablespoon hoisin sauce

- 1 tablespoon sesame oil

- 2 cloves garlic, minced

- 1 teaspoon ginger, grated

- Cooked brown rice for serving

Instructions:

1. In a bowl, marinate sliced beef in soy sauce, oyster sauce, and sesame oil for 10 minutes.

2. Heat a wok or skillet over high heat. Stir-fry beef until browned, then remove from the pan.

3. In the same pan, stir-fry broccoli and bell pepper until crisp-tender.

4. Add minced garlic and grated ginger, stir briefly.

5. Return cooked beef to the pan, toss everything together, and serve over brown rice.

6. Lemon Herb Grilled Chicken Wrap

Description: Revitalize your lunch with these lemon herb grilled chicken wraps. Tender grilled chicken meets crisp veggies, all wrapped in a whole-grain tortilla for a delightful and portable meal.

Serving Size: 2 wraps

Prep Time: 15 minutes

Cooking Time: 10 minutes

Ingredients:

- 2 boneless, skinless chicken breasts

- Zest and juice of 1 lemon

- 1 tablespoon olive oil

- 1 teaspoon dried oregano

- Salt and pepper to taste

- 2 whole-grain tortillas

- Greek yogurt or tzatziki sauce

- Sliced cucumber, tomato, and red onion

- Fresh dill for garnish

Instructions:

1. In a bowl, mix lemon zest, lemon juice, olive oil, dried oregano, salt, and pepper.

2. Marinate chicken breasts in the lemon herb mixture for 10 minutes.

3. Grill chicken until cooked through, then slice into strips.

4. Warm tortillas and spread Greek yogurt or tzatziki sauce.

5. Fill each tortilla with grilled chicken, sliced cucumber, tomato, red onion, and garnish with fresh dill.

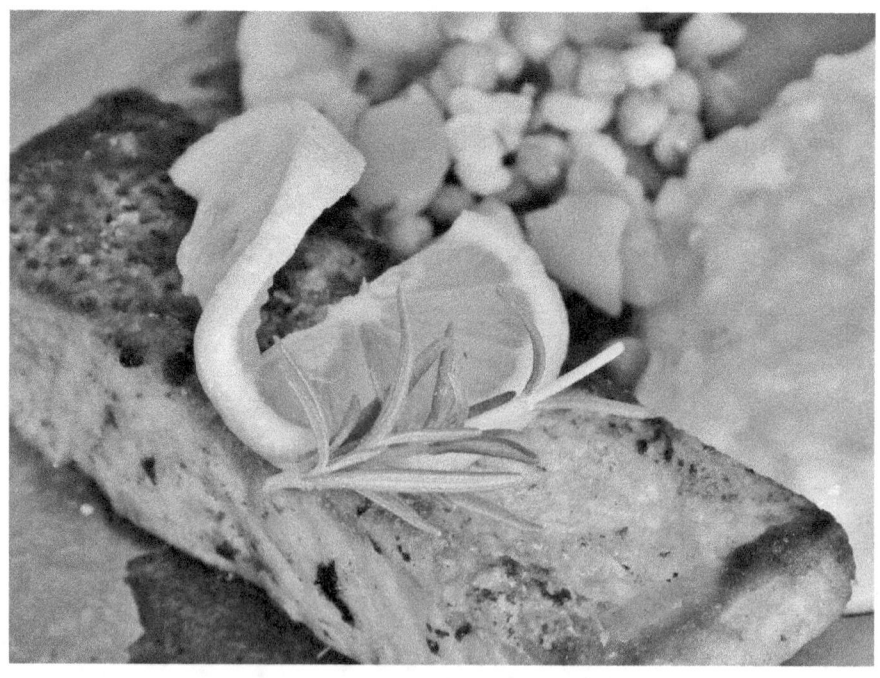

7. Spaghetti Squash with Pesto and Cherry Tomatoes

Description: Swap traditional pasta for nutrient-rich spaghetti squash in this light and flavorful dish. Tossed with homemade pesto and cherry tomatoes, it's a guilt-free lunch option.

Serving Size: 2 servings

Prep Time: 15 minutes

Cooking Time: 40 minutes

Ingredients:

- 1 medium spaghetti squash, halved and seeds removed

- 2 cups fresh basil leaves

- 1/2 cup pine nuts

- 1/2 cup grated Parmesan cheese

- 2 cloves garlic

- 1/2 cup extra virgin olive oil

- Salt and pepper to taste

- Cherry tomatoes, halved, for topping

Instructions:

1. Preheat the oven to 375°F (190°C).

2. Place spaghetti squash halves on a baking sheet, cut side down. Bake for 30-40 minutes until tender.

3. In a food processor, blend basil, pine nuts, Parmesan, garlic, olive oil, salt, and pepper to make pesto.

4. Scrape spaghetti squash with a fork to create "noodles."

5. Toss spaghetti squash noodles with pesto and top with halved cherry tomatoes.

8. Black Bean and Quinoa Burrito Bowl

Description: Build your own nutritious burrito bowl with this black bean and quinoa creation. Packed with protein and fiber, it's a wholesome lunch that satisfies your taste buds.

Serving Size: 2 servings

Prep Time: 20 minutes

Cooking Time: 15 minutes

Ingredients:

- 1 cup quinoa, cooked

- 1 can (15 oz) black beans, drained and rinsed

- 1 cup corn kernels (fresh or frozen)

- 1 avocado, sliced

- 1/2 cup cherry tomatoes, halved

- Fresh cilantro for garnish

- Lime wedges for squeezing

- Optional: Salsa or hot sauce

Instructions:

1. In bowls, layer cooked quinoa, black beans, corn, avocado, and cherry tomatoes.

2. Garnish with fresh cilantro and serve with lime wedges.

3. Optional: Add salsa or hot sauce for extra flavor.

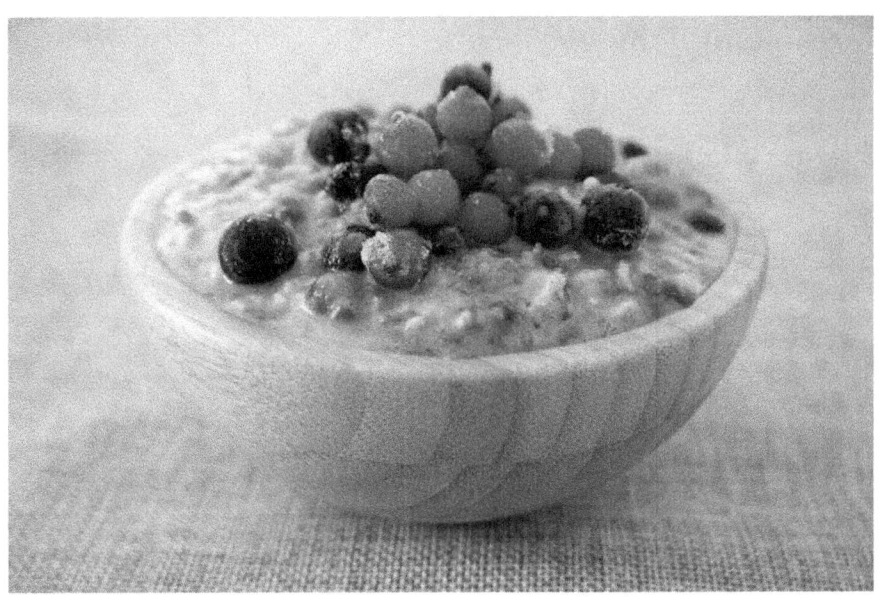

9. Sweet Potato and Chickpea Buddha Bowl

Description: Embrace the Buddha bowl trend with this nourishing combination of roasted sweet potatoes, chickpeas, and a variety of colorful veggies. Drizzle with tahini for a finishing touch.

Serving Size: 2 servings

Prep Time: 20 minutes

Cooking Time: 30 minutes

Ingredients:

- 2 medium sweet potatoes, peeled and cubed

- 1 can (15 oz) chickpeas, drained and rinsed

- 1 tablespoon olive oil

- 1 teaspoon cumin

- 1 teaspoon paprika

- Salt and pepper to taste

- Mixed greens for the base

- Cherry tomatoes, cucumber, and red onion for topping

- Tahini dressing

Instructions:

1. Preheat the oven to 400°F (200°C).

2. Toss sweet potatoes and chickpeas with olive oil, cumin, paprika, salt, and pepper.

3. Roast in the oven for 25-30 minutes until golden and crisp.

4. Assemble Buddha bowls with mixed greens, roasted sweet potatoes, chickpeas, and fresh veggies.

5. Drizzle with tahini dressing before serving.

10. Lentil and Vegetable Soup

Description: Warm up your afternoon with a hearty lentil and vegetable soup. Packed with protein, fiber, and an array of colorful veggies, it's a comforting and nutritious lunch option.

Serving Size: 4 servings

Prep Time: 15 minutes

Cooking Time: 30 minutes

Ingredients:

- 1 cup dried green lentils, rinsed

- 1 onion, chopped

- 2 carrots, diced

- 2 celery stalks, chopped

- 3 cloves garlic, minced

- 1 can (14 oz) diced tomatoes

- 6 cups vegetable broth

- 1 teaspoon cumin

- 1 teaspoon coriander

- 1 bay leaf

- Salt and pepper to taste

- Fresh parsley for garnish

Instructions:

1. In a large pot, sauté onion, carrots, and celery until softened.

2. Add minced garlic and sauté for an additional minute.

3. Pour in diced tomatoes, vegetable broth, lentils, cumin, coriander, bay leaf, salt, and pepper.

4. Bring to a boil, then reduce heat and simmer for 25-30 minutes.

5. Garnish with fresh parsley before serving.

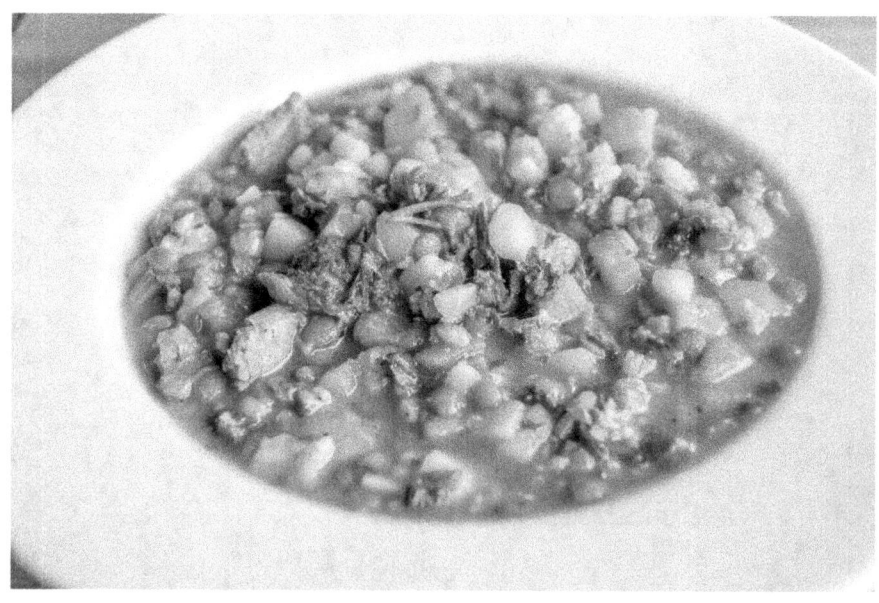

Dinner Sensations: Indulge in Healing Dinners

Here are 10 dinner recipes from "Anti-Inflammatory Diet," designed to delight your taste buds and provide a nourishing end to your day:

1. Lemon Herb Baked Salmon

Description: Savor the simplicity and freshness of this lemon herb baked salmon. The combination of zesty lemon, aromatic herbs, and perfectly baked salmon fillets creates a dinner sensation that's both elegant and easy to prepare.

Serving Size: 2 servings

Prep Time: 10 minutes

Cooking Time: 20 minutes

Ingredients:

- 2 salmon fillets

- Zest and juice of 1 lemon

- 2 tablespoons olive oil

- 2 cloves garlic, minced

- 1 teaspoon dried dill

- Salt and pepper to taste

- Fresh parsley for garnish

Instructions:

1. Preheat the oven to 400°F (200°C).

2. In a bowl, mix lemon zest, lemon juice, olive oil, minced garlic, dried dill, salt, and pepper.

3. Place salmon fillets on a baking sheet, pour the lemon herb mixture over them.

4. Bake for 20 minutes or until salmon flakes easily with a fork.

5. Garnish with fresh parsley before serving.

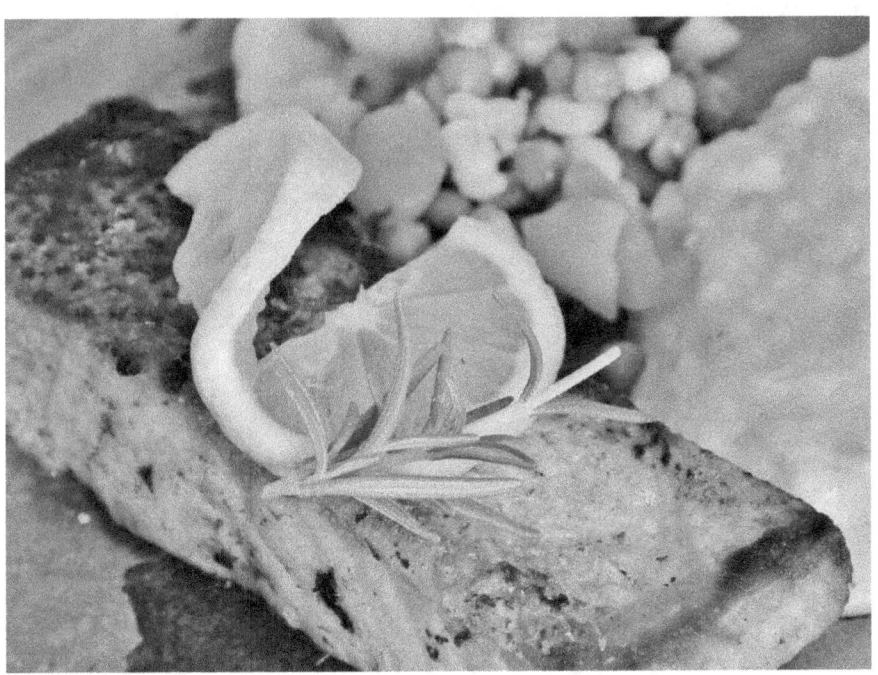

2. Vegetarian Cauliflower and Chickpea Curry

Description: Indulge in a flavorful vegetarian curry that combines the nuttiness of chickpeas with the delicate texture of cauliflower. This curry is a celebration of spices, creating a satisfying and wholesome dinner.

Serving Size: 4 servings

Prep Time: 15 minutes

Cooking Time: 25 minutes

Ingredients:

- 1 cauliflower, cut into florets

- 1 can (15 oz) chickpeas, drained and rinsed

- 1 onion, finely chopped

- 2 cloves garlic, minced

- 1 can (14 oz) diced tomatoes

- 1 can (14 oz) coconut milk

- 2 tablespoons curry powder

- 1 teaspoon ground cumin

- 1 teaspoon ground coriander

- Salt and pepper to taste

- Fresh cilantro for garnish

Instructions:

1. In a large pot, sauté chopped onion and garlic until softened.

2. Add cauliflower florets, chickpeas, diced tomatoes, coconut milk, curry powder, cumin, coriander, salt, and pepper.

3. Simmer for 20-25 minutes until cauliflower is tender.

4. Garnish with fresh cilantro and serve over rice or quinoa.

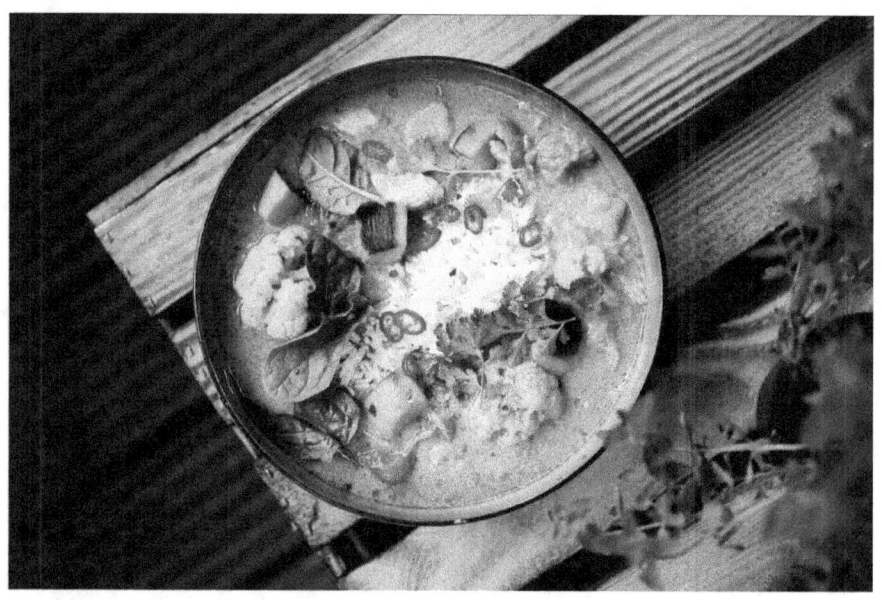

3. Balsamic Glazed Chicken with Roasted Vegetables

Description: Elevate your dinner with this balsamic glazed chicken paired with a colorful medley of roasted vegetables. The sweet and tangy glaze adds a delightful touch to this satisfying and visually appealing dish.

Serving Size: 2 servings

Prep Time: 15 minutes

Cooking Time: 30 minutes

Ingredients:

- 2 boneless, skinless chicken breasts

- 1 cup cherry tomatoes, halved

- 1 bell pepper, sliced

- 1 zucchini, sliced

- 2 tablespoons balsamic glaze

- 2 tablespoons olive oil

- 1 teaspoon dried oregano

- Salt and pepper to taste

- Fresh basil for garnish

Instructions:

1. Preheat the oven to 400°F (200°C).

2. Season chicken breasts with salt, pepper, and dried oregano.

3. In a bowl, toss cherry tomatoes, bell pepper, and zucchini with olive oil, salt, and pepper.

4. Place chicken and vegetables on a baking sheet. Drizzle balsamic glaze over the chicken.

5. Roast for 25-30 minutes or until chicken is cooked through.

6. Garnish with fresh basil before serving.

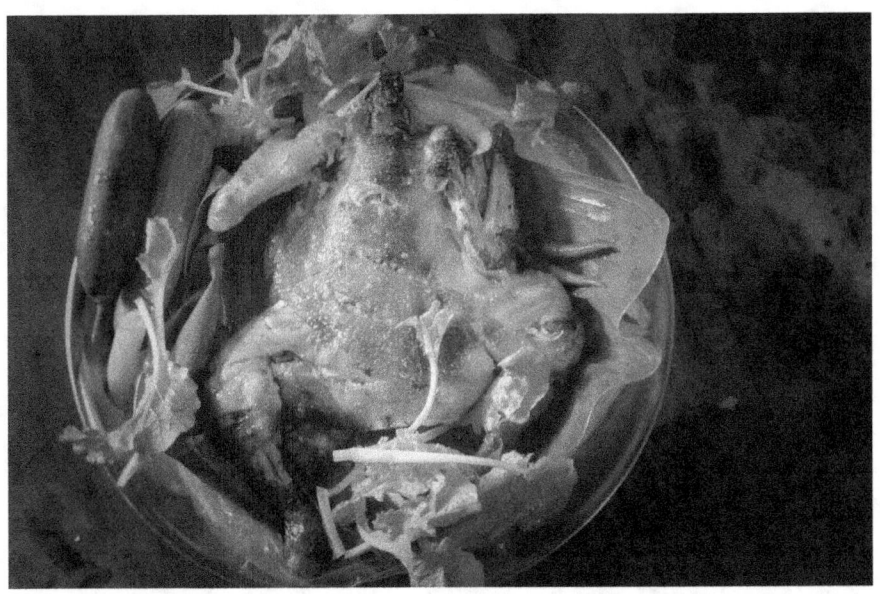

4. Quinoa and Black Bean Stuffed Bell Peppers

Description: Experience a dinner sensation with these quinoa and black bean stuffed bell peppers. Packed with protein, fiber, and vibrant flavors, they make for a satisfying and wholesome meal.

Serving Size: 4 servings

Prep Time: 20 minutes

Cooking Time: 30 minutes

Ingredients:

- 4 bell peppers, halved and seeds removed

- 1 cup quinoa, cooked

- 1 can (15 oz) black beans, drained and rinsed

- 1 cup corn kernels (fresh or frozen)

- 1 cup cherry tomatoes, diced

- 1/2 cup red onion, finely chopped

- 1 cup shredded cheddar cheese

- 1 teaspoon cumin

- 1 teaspoon chili powder

- Salt and pepper to taste

- Fresh cilantro for garnish

Instructions:

1. Preheat the oven to 375°F (190°C).

2. In a large bowl, mix cooked quinoa, black beans, corn, cherry tomatoes, red onion, shredded cheddar, cumin, chili powder, salt, and pepper.

3. Stuff bell pepper halves with the quinoa mixture.

4. Bake for 25-30 minutes or until peppers are tender.

5. Garnish with fresh cilantro and serve.

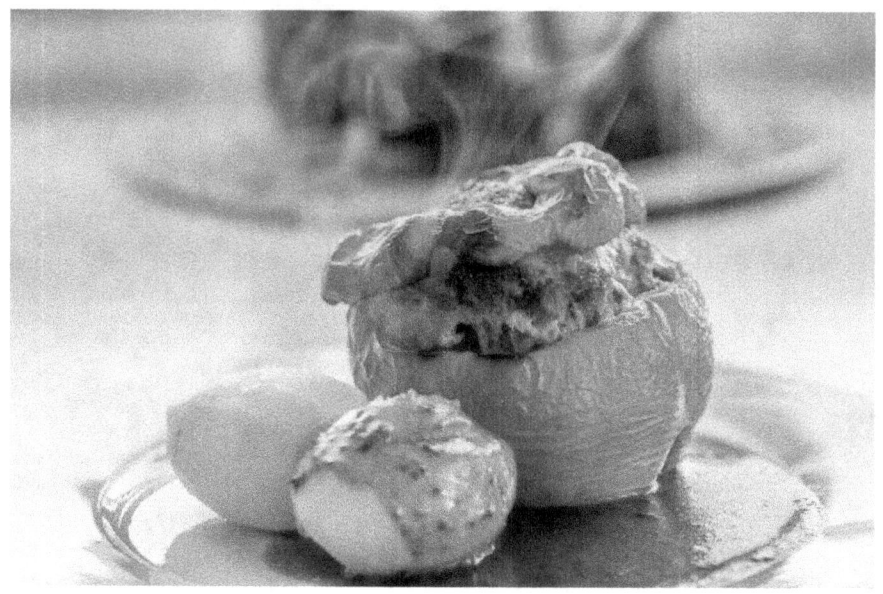

5. Garlic Butter Shrimp with Asparagus

Description: Elevate your dinner with this garlic butter shrimp paired with crisp asparagus. The simplicity of this dish allows the natural flavors to shine, creating a delightful and quick-to-make sensation.

Serving Size: 2 servings

Prep Time: 10 minutes

Cooking Time: 10 minutes

Ingredients:

- 1 lb large shrimp, peeled and deveined

- 1 bunch asparagus, trimmed

- 4 tablespoons unsalted butter

- 4 cloves garlic, minced

- Juice of 1 lemon

- Salt and pepper to taste

- Fresh parsley for garnish

Instructions:

1. In a skillet, melt butter over medium heat. Add minced garlic and sauté until fragrant.

2. Add shrimp and cook until pink, about 2-3 minutes per side.

3. Add asparagus to the skillet and cook until tender-crisp.

4. Squeeze lemon juice over the shrimp and asparagus. Season with salt and pepper.

5. Garnish with fresh parsley and serve.

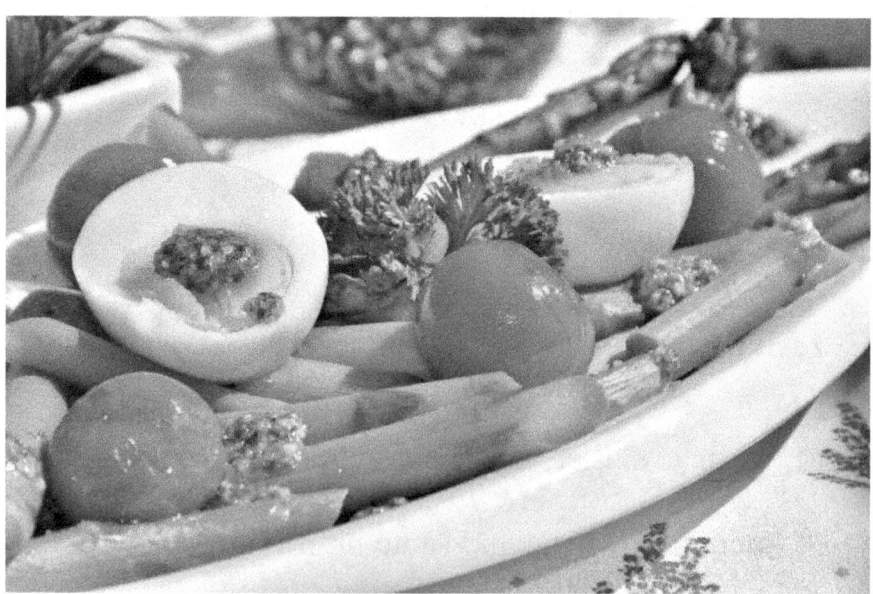

6. Eggplant Parmesan

Description: Indulge in the comforting flavors of this classic eggplant Parmesan. Layers of thinly sliced eggplant, rich marinara sauce, and melted cheese create a dinner sensation that's both hearty and satisfying.

Serving Size: 4 servings

Prep Time: 30 minutes

Cooking Time: 30 minutes

Ingredients:

- 2 large eggplants, sliced

- 2 cups marinara sauce

- 2 cups shredded mozzarella cheese

- 1 cup grated Parmesan cheese

- 1 cup breadcrumbs

- 2 eggs, beaten

- 1 teaspoon dried oregano

- 1 teaspoon dried basil

- Salt and pepper to taste

- Fresh basil for garnish

Instructions:

1. Preheat the oven to 375°F (190°C).

2. Dip eggplant slices in beaten eggs, then coat with breadcrumbs seasoned with dried oregano, dried basil, salt, and pepper.

3. In a baking dish, layer marinara sauce, eggplant slices, mozzarella, and Parmesan. Repeat.

4. Bake for 25-30 minutes or until the cheese is melted and bubbly.

5. Garnish with fresh basil before serving.

7. Spinach and Feta Stuffed Chicken Breast

Description: Elevate your dinner with these spinach and feta stuffed chicken breasts. The combination of tender chicken, flavorful spinach, and creamy feta creates a delicious and visually appealing dish.

Serving Size: 2 servings

Prep Time: 15 minutes

Cooking Time: 25 minutes

Ingredients:

- 2 boneless, skinless chicken breasts

- 2 cups fresh spinach, chopped

- 1/2 cup feta cheese, crumbled

- 2 cloves garlic, minced

- 1 teaspoon dried oregano

- Salt and pepper to taste

- Olive oil for cooking

- Lemon wedges for serving

Instructions:

1. Preheat the oven to 375°F (190°C).

2. In a bowl, mix chopped spinach, crumbled feta, minced garlic, dried oregano, salt, and pepper.

3. Cut a pocket into each chicken breast and stuff with the spinach and feta mixture.

4. Secure with toothpicks and season the outside with salt and pepper.

5. In a skillet, heat olive oil over medium-high heat. Sear chicken on each side until golden.

6. Transfer chicken to the oven and bake for 20 minutes or until cooked through.

7. Serve with lemon wedges for squeezing.

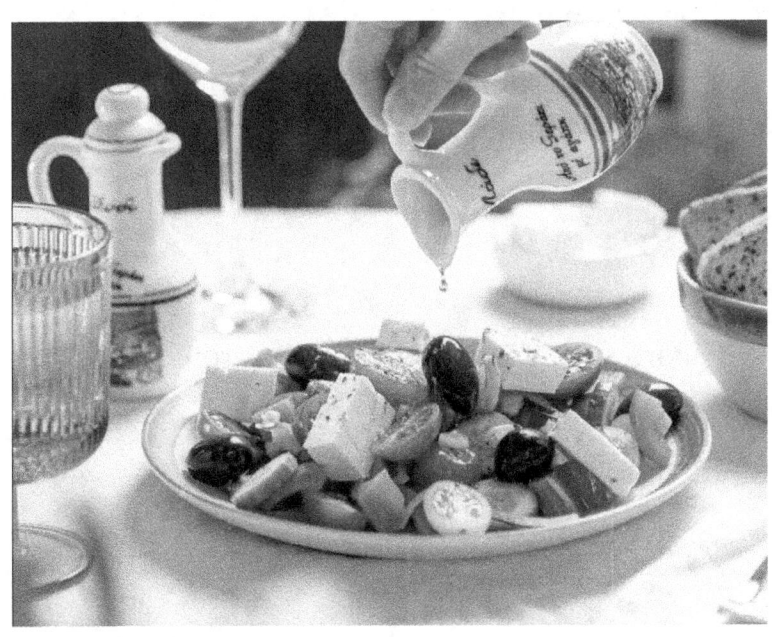

8. Mushroom and Quinoa Stuffed Acorn Squash

Description: Enjoy a dinner sensation with these mushroom and quinoa stuffed acorn squash. The nutty quinoa and savory mushroom filling complement the natural sweetness of acorn squash for a wholesome and flavorful dish.

Serving Size: 4 servings

Prep Time: 20 minutes

Cooking Time: 40 minutes

Ingredients:

- 2 acorn squash, halved and seeds removed

- 1 cup quinoa, cooked

- 2 cups cremini mushrooms, chopped

- 1 onion, finely chopped

- 2 cloves garlic, minced

- 1 teaspoon thyme

- 1/2 cup grated Gruyere cheese

- Olive oil for cooking

- Salt and pepper to taste

- Fresh parsley for garnish

Instructions:

1. Preheat the oven to 375°F (190°C).

2. Place acorn squash halves on a baking sheet, cut side down. Bake for 30 minutes.

3. In a skillet, sauté chopped onion and garlic until softened.

4. Add mushrooms and cook until browned. Stir in cooked quinoa, thyme, salt, and pepper.

5. Stuff each acorn squash half with the quinoa and mushroom mixture.

6. Top with grated Gruyere and bake for an additional 10 minutes or until cheese is melted.

7. Garnish with fresh parsley before serving.

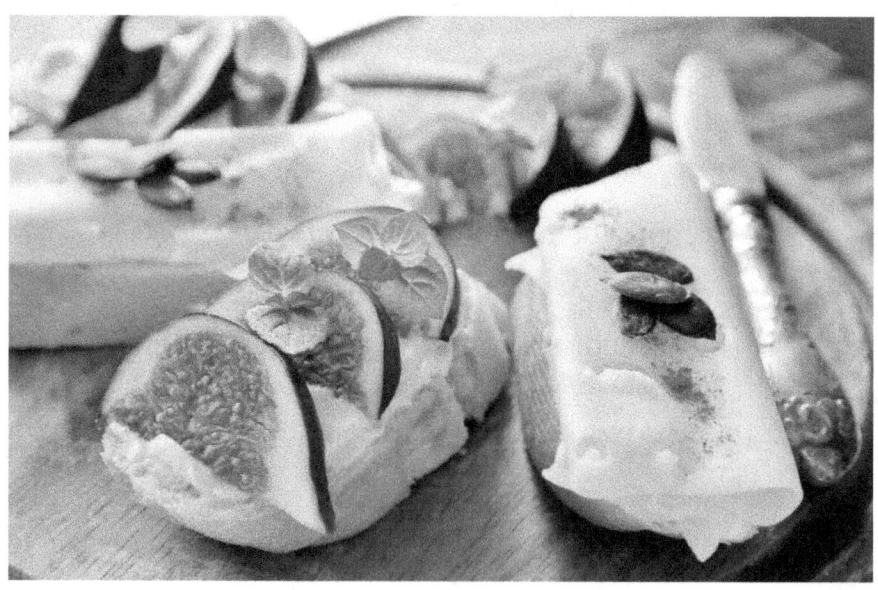

Snack Attack: Healthy Bites for Every Craving

Here are 10 healthy and satisfying snack recipes from "Anti-Inflammatory Diet" that cater to various cravings:

1. Energy-Boosting Protein Balls

Description: Revitalize your energy with these protein-packed balls. Packed with nuts, seeds, and a touch of sweetness, they're the perfect snack to keep you going.

Serving Size: 12 balls

Prep Time: 15 minutes

Ingredients:

- 1 cup rolled oats

- 1/2 cup almond butter

- 1/3 cup honey or maple syrup

- 1/2 cup protein powder

- 1/4 cup chia seeds

- 1/4 cup dark chocolate chips

- 1 teaspoon vanilla extract

- Pinch of salt

Instructions:

1. In a bowl, mix all ingredients until well combined.

2. Roll the mixture into bite-sized balls.

3. Place in the refrigerator for at least 30 minutes to set.

2. Greek Yogurt Parfait with Berries

Description: Indulge in a parfait that's as pleasing to the eyes as it is to your taste buds. Layers of Greek yogurt, fresh berries, and crunchy granola create a snack that's both delicious and nutritious.

Serving Size: 1 parfait

Prep Time: 5 minutes

Ingredients:

- 1 cup Greek yogurt

- 1/2 cup mixed berries (strawberries, blueberries, raspberries)

- 1/4 cup granola

- Drizzle of honey for sweetness

Instructions:

1. In a glass or bowl, layer Greek yogurt, mixed berries, and granola.

2. Repeat the layers until you reach the top.

3. Drizzle honey on top for extra sweetness.

3. Avocado and Chickpea Toast

Description: Upgrade your toast game with this creamy and satisfying avocado and chickpea spread. Packed with healthy fats and protein, it's a snack that keeps you satisfied.

Serving Size: 2 toasts

Prep Time: 10 minutes

Ingredients:

- 1 ripe avocado

- 1/2 cup canned chickpeas, drained and rinsed

- 1 tablespoon lemon juice

- Salt and pepper to taste

- 2 slices whole-grain bread

- Optional toppings: cherry tomatoes, radish slices, microgreens

Instructions:

1. In a bowl, mash the avocado and chickpeas together.

2. Add lemon juice, salt, and pepper. Mix well.

3. Toast the bread slices.

4. Spread the avocado and chickpea mixture on the toasted bread.

5. Top with cherry tomatoes, radish slices, or microgreens if desired.

4. Cucumber and Hummus Roll-Ups

Description: Refresh your snack time with these light and crunchy cucumber roll-ups. Filled with hummus and veggies, they make for a hydrating and satisfying bite.

Serving Size: 4 roll-ups

Prep Time: 10 minutes

Ingredients:

- 1 large cucumber

- 1/2 cup hummus

- 1/4 cup thinly sliced bell peppers

- 1/4 cup shredded carrots

- Fresh dill for garnish

Instructions:

1. Slice the cucumber lengthwise into thin strips using a peeler.

2. Spread hummus evenly on each cucumber strip.

3. Place sliced bell peppers and shredded carrots along one edge.

4. Roll up the cucumber strip with the veggies inside.

5. Secure with a toothpick and garnish with fresh dill.

5. Homemade Trail Mix

Description: Create your personalized trail mix for a snack that's both satisfying and customizable. A mix of nuts, seeds, dried fruits, and a hint of chocolate hits all the right notes.

Serving Size: 1 cup

Prep Time: 5 minutes

Ingredients:

- 1/4 cup almonds

- 1/4 cup walnuts

- 1/4 cup pumpkin seeds

- 1/4 cup dried cranberries

- 2 tablespoons dark chocolate chips

- 2 tablespoons coconut flakes

Instructions:

1. In a bowl, mix all the ingredients together.

2. Portion into small snack-sized bags for convenience.

6. Caprese Skewers

Description: Enjoy the classic Caprese salad in a bite-sized form. These skewers with cherry tomatoes, fresh mozzarella, and basil are a refreshing and satisfying snack.

Serving Size: 4 skewers

Prep Time: 10 minutes

Ingredients:

- 1 cup cherry tomatoes

- 1 cup fresh mozzarella balls

- Fresh basil leaves

- Balsamic glaze for drizzling

Instructions:

1. Thread a cherry tomato, a mozzarella ball, and a basil leaf onto each skewer.

2. Arrange on a serving plate and drizzle with balsamic glaze before serving.

7. Sweet Potato Chips with Guacamole

Description: Swap traditional potato chips for these baked sweet potato chips. Paired with homemade guacamole, it's a crunchy and creamy snack that satisfies your craving.

Serving Size: 1 cup chips, 1/2 cup guacamole

Prep Time: 20 minutes

Ingredients:

- 1 large sweet potato, thinly sliced

- 1 tablespoon olive oil

- 1/2 teaspoon paprika

- Salt and pepper to taste

- For guacamole: 2 ripe avocados, 1 clove garlic (minced), 1 lime (juiced), salt, and pepper

Instructions:

1. Preheat the oven to 400°F (200°C).

2. Toss sweet potato slices with olive oil, paprika, salt, and pepper.

3. Arrange in a single layer on a baking sheet and bake for 15-20 minutes or until crispy.

4. While the chips are baking, mash avocados for guacamole and mix with minced garlic, lime juice, salt, and pepper.

5. Serve sweet potato chips with guacamole.

8. Spicy Edamame

Description: Add a kick to your snack routine with these spicy edamame beans. Satisfyingly crunchy and rich in protein, they make for a flavorful and addictive snack.

Serving Size: 1 cup

Prep Time: 5 minutes

Ingredients:

- 2 cups edamame (thawed if frozen)

- 1 tablespoon soy sauce

- 1 teaspoon sesame oil

- 1/2 teaspoon chili flakes

- 1 teaspoon sesame seeds

Instructions:

1. In a bowl, toss edamame with soy sauce, sesame oil, and chili flakes.

2. Microwave or steam edamame until heated through.

3. Sprinkle with sesame

seeds before serving.

9. Roasted Chickpeas Three Ways

Description: Transform simple chickpeas into a crunchy and satisfying snack with these three flavor variations. Choose from savory, sweet, or spicy to suit your cravings.

Serving Size: 1 cup each flavor

Prep Time: 10 minutes

Cooking Time: 40 minutes

Ingredients: For Savory:

- 1 can (15 oz) chickpeas, drained and rinsed

- 1 tablespoon olive oil

- 1 teaspoon smoked paprika

- 1/2 teaspoon garlic powder

- Salt to taste

For Sweet:

- 1 can (15 oz) chickpeas, drained and rinsed

- 1 tablespoon coconut oil, melted

- 1 tablespoon honey or maple syrup

- 1 teaspoon cinnamon

- Pinch of salt

For Spicy:

- 1 can (15 oz) chickpeas, drained and rinsed

- 1 tablespoon olive oil

- 1 teaspoon chili powder

- 1/2 teaspoon cumin

- Salt to taste

Instructions:

1. Preheat the oven to 400°F (200°C).

2. Rinse and dry chickpeas thoroughly.

3. For each flavor variation, mix chickpeas with the specified ingredients in a bowl.

4. Spread chickpeas in a single layer on a baking sheet.

5. Bake for 30-40 minutes or until crispy, shaking the pan halfway through.

10. Stuffed Bell Pepper Poppers

Description: Elevate the classic stuffed pepper concept into bite-sized poppers. Filled with a mix of cream cheese, veggies, and a hint of spice, these poppers make for a delightful and shareable snack.

Serving Size: 12 poppers

Prep Time: 20 minutes

Cooking Time: 15 minutes

Ingredients:

- 6 mini bell peppers, halved and seeds removed

- 1/2 cup cream cheese, softened

- 1/4 cup diced tomatoes

- 1/4 cup diced cucumber

- 1/4 cup diced red onion

- 1 jalapeño, finely chopped (optional for spice)

- Fresh cilantro for garnish

Instructions:

1. Preheat the oven to 375°F (190°C).

2. In a bowl, mix cream cheese, diced tomatoes, diced cucumber, diced red onion, and chopped jalapeño.

3. Fill each mini bell pepper half with the cream cheese mixture.

4. Place on a baking sheet and bake for 15 minutes or until the peppers are tender.

5. Garnish with fresh cilantro before serving.

Enjoy these flavorful and nourishing snack recipes to satisfy your cravings!

Decadent Desserts: Sweets Without Sacrifice

Here are 10 decadent dessert recipes from "Anti-Inflammatory Diet" that offer sweet indulgence without sacrifice:

1. Dark Chocolate Avocado Mousse

Description: Experience the richness of chocolate combined with the creamy texture of avocado in this guilt-free mousse. It's a delightful dessert that satisfies your sweet tooth while providing a dose of healthy fats.

Serving Size: 4 servings

Prep Time: 15 minutes

Ingredients:

- 2 ripe avocados

- 1/2 cup dark cocoa powder

- 1/4 cup maple syrup or honey

- 1 teaspoon vanilla extract

- Pinch of salt

- Fresh berries for garnish

Instructions:

1. In a blender, combine avocados, cocoa powder, maple syrup, vanilla extract, and a pinch of salt.

2. Blend until smooth and creamy.

3. Divide the mousse into serving glasses.

4. Chill in the refrigerator for at least 1 hour.

5. Garnish with fresh berries before serving.

2. Coconut Chia Seed Pudding

Description: Indulge in a luscious coconut chia seed pudding that's both sweet and satisfying. The combination of coconut milk and chia seeds creates a creamy texture, making it a delightful guilt-free dessert.

Serving Size: 2 servings

Prep Time: 10 minutes

Ingredients:

- 1 can (14 oz) coconut milk

- 1/4 cup chia seeds

- 2 tablespoons maple syrup or agave syrup

- 1/2 teaspoon vanilla extract

- Fresh mango slices for topping

Instructions:

1. In a bowl, whisk together coconut milk, chia seeds, maple syrup, and vanilla extract.

2. Let the mixture sit for 5 minutes, then whisk again to prevent clumps.

3. Refrigerate for at least 4 hours or overnight.

4. Spoon the chia pudding into serving bowls.

5. Top with fresh mango slices before serving.

3. Almond Butter Banana Oat Bars

Description: These almond butter banana oat bars are a wholesome and decadent treat. Packed with natural sweetness from bananas and a nutty flavor from almond butter, they make for a delightful dessert or snack.

Serving Size: 8 bars

Prep Time: 15 minutes

Cooking Time: 25 minutes

Ingredients:

- 2 ripe bananas, mashed

- 1/2 cup almond butter

- 1/4 cup honey or maple syrup

- 1 teaspoon vanilla extract

- 2 cups rolled oats

- 1/2 teaspoon baking powder

- Pinch of salt

- Dark chocolate chips for topping

Instructions:

1. Preheat the oven to 350°F (175°C). Grease a baking dish.

2. In a bowl, mix mashed bananas, almond butter, honey, and vanilla extract.

3. Add rolled oats, baking powder, and a pinch of salt. Mix until well combined.

4. Press the mixture into the prepared baking dish.

5. Sprinkle dark chocolate chips on top.

6. Bake for 25 minutes or until the edges are golden brown.

7. Allow to cool before cutting into bars.

4. Raspberry Almond Chia Pudding Parfait

Description: Elevate your dessert experience with this delightful raspberry almond chia pudding parfait. Layers of almond chia pudding and fresh raspberries create a visually appealing and flavorful treat.

Serving Size: 2 parfaits

Prep Time: 15 minutes

Ingredients:

- 1 can (14 oz) coconut milk

- 1/4 cup chia seeds

- 2 tablespoons almond butter

- 2 tablespoons maple syrup

- 1/2 teaspoon almond extract

- Fresh raspberries for layering

- Sliced almonds for garnish

Instructions:

1. In a bowl, whisk together coconut milk, chia seeds, almond butter, maple syrup, and almond extract.

2. Refrigerate for at least 4 hours or overnight.

3. Layer the chia pudding and fresh raspberries in serving glasses.

4. Repeat the layers until you reach the top.

5. Garnish with sliced almonds before serving.

5. Baked Apple Crisp with Pecan Topping

Description: Indulge in the comforting flavors of baked apple crisp without the guilt. This version features a nutty pecan topping that adds a delightful crunch to every bite.

Serving Size: 6 servings

Prep Time: 20 minutes

Cooking Time: 40 minutes

Ingredients:

- 4 apples, peeled, cored, and sliced

- 1 tablespoon lemon juice

- 2 tablespoons maple syrup

- 1 teaspoon ground cinnamon

- 1/2 teaspoon nutmeg

- Pinch of salt

- 1 cup rolled oats

- 1/2 cup chopped pecans

- 1/4 cup coconut oil, melted

- 2 tablespoons maple syrup

Instructions:

1. Preheat the oven to 350°F (175°C). Grease a baking dish.

2. In a bowl, toss sliced apples with lemon juice, maple syrup, cinnamon, nutmeg, and a pinch of salt.

3. Spread the apples evenly in the baking dish.

4. In another bowl, mix rolled oats, chopped pecans, melted coconut oil, and maple syrup.

5. Sprinkle the oat mixture over the apples.

6. Bake for 40 minutes or until the top is golden brown.

7. Allow to cool slightly before serving.

6. Chocolate-Dipped Strawberries with Pistachios

Description: Elevate the classic chocolate-dipped strawberries with a sprinkle of pistachios. This simple yet decadent dessert is perfect for special occasions or a sweet treat anytime.

Serving Size: 12 strawberries

Prep Time: 15 minutes

Ingredients:

- 12 fresh strawberries, washed and dried

- 4 oz dark chocolate, melted

- 1/4 cup chopped pistachios

Instructions:

1. Line a tray with parchment paper.

2. Dip each strawberry into melted dark chocolate, covering about two-thirds of the fruit.

3. Place the dipped strawberries on the parchment paper.

4. Sprinkle chopped pistachios over the chocolate.

5. Allow the chocolate to set before serving.

7. Banana Bread Mug Cake

Description: Satisfy your banana bread cravings in minutes with this easy and delicious banana bread mug cake. It's a single-serving dessert that's perfect for a quick indulgence.

Serving Size: 1 mug cake

Prep Time: 5 minutes

Cooking Time: 2 minutes

Ingredients:

- 1 ripe banana, mashed

- 2 tablespoons almond flour

- 1 tablespoon coconut flour

- 1/2 teaspoon baking powder

- 1/4 teaspoon cinnamon

- 1 egg

- 1 tablespoon maple syrup

- 1/2 teaspoon vanilla extract

Instructions:

1. In a microwave-safe mug, combine mashed banana, almond flour, coconut flour, baking powder, and cinnamon.

2. Add the egg, maple syrup, and vanilla extract. Mix well.

3. Microwave on high for 2 minutes or until the cake is set.

4. Allow to cool slightly before enjoying.

8. Mango Coconut Rice Pudding

Description: Transport yourself to a tropical paradise with this mango coconut rice pudding. Creamy coconut milk, fragrant mango, and tender rice create a dessert that's both exotic and comforting.

Serving Size: 4 servings

Prep Time: 10 minutes

Cooking Time: 25 minutes

Ingredients:

- 1 cup arborio rice

- 1 can (14 oz) coconut milk

- 1/4 cup honey or agave syrup

- 1/2 teaspoon vanilla extract

- 1 ripe mango, diced

- Toasted coconut flakes for garnish

Instructions:

1. In a saucepan, combine arborio rice, coconut milk, honey, and vanilla extract.

2. Bring to a simmer over medium heat, then reduce heat to low and cover.

3. Cook for 20-25 minutes, stirring occasionally, until the rice is tender and the pudding has thickened.

4. Stir in diced mango.

5. Divide into serving bowls and garnish with toasted coconut flakes.

9. Cinnamon Baked Pears with Walnuts

Description: Experience the warm and comforting flavors of cinnamon baked pears. This simple dessert features sweet pears, a hint of cinnamon, and crunchy walnuts for a delightful treat.

Serving Size: 4 servings

Prep Time: 10 minutes

Cooking Time: 20 minutes

Ingredients:

- 4 ripe pears, halved and cored

- 2 tablespoons melted coconut oil

- 2 tablespoons maple syrup

- 1 teaspoon ground cinnamon

- 1/4 cup chopped walnuts

Instructions:

1. Preheat the oven to 375°F (190°C). Grease a baking dish.

2. Place pear halves in the baking dish.

3. In a small bowl, mix melted coconut oil, maple syrup, and ground cinnamon.

4. Brush the mixture over the pears.

5. Sprinkle chopped walnuts on top.

6. Bake for 20 minutes or until the pears are tender.

7. Serve warm.

10. Blueberry Almond Tart with Oat Crust

Description: Indulge in a delicious blueberry almond tart with an oat crust. This dessert combines the sweetness of blueberries with the nutty flavor of almonds for a delightful and visually appealing treat.

Serving Size: 8 slices

Prep Time: 20 minutes

Cooking Time: 25 minutes

Ingredients: For the crust:

- 1 cup rolled oats

- 1/2 cup almond flour

- 1/4 cup melted coconut oil

- 2 tablespoons maple syrup

- Pinch of salt

For the filling:

- 2 cups fresh blueberries

- 1/2 cup almond meal

- 1/4 cup maple syrup

- 1 teaspoon vanilla extract

- Sliced almonds for garnish

Instructions: For the crust:

1. Preheat the oven to 350°F (175°C). Grease a tart pan.

2. In a food processor, blend rolled oats until they form coarse flour.

3. In a bowl, mix oat flour, almond flour, melted coconut oil, maple syrup, and a pinch of salt.

4. Press the mixture into the tart pan, forming an even crust.

5. Bake for 10 minutes or until golden brown.

For the filling:

1. In a bowl, combine fresh blueberries, almond meal, maple syrup, and vanilla extract.

2. Spoon the blueberry mixture onto the baked crust.

3. Bake for an additional 15 minutes.

4. Garnish with sliced almonds before serving.

Enjoy these decadent desserts that bring sweetness without sacrifice!

CHAPTER SIX

Mindful Eating Practices

The Connection Between Mindfulness and Health

Welcome to the transformative journey of Chapter 6, where the profound link between mindfulness and your well-being comes to light. Beyond the mere act of eating, mindful eating fosters a connection between your mind and body, creating a harmony that extends far beyond the dining table.

In the intricate dance of life, mindfulness becomes a guiding force. Studies have shown that embracing mindfulness in your eating habits can have a profound impact on your overall health. As you savor each bite with awareness, you not only nourish your body but also cultivate a deeper understanding of your relationship with food.

Practical Tips for Mindful Eating

Embark on a practical exploration of mindful eating with actionable tips that breathe life into this holistic practice. As you dive into your meals, consider the textures, flavors, and aromas that unfold with each culinary experience. Mindful eating is not a rigid set of rules but an art to be cultivated.

1. **Engage Your Senses:** Allow the vibrant symphony of colors, scents, and tastes to captivate your senses. Observe the interplay of textures as you savor each bite mindfully.

2. **Slow Down and Savor:** In a world that often rushes, mindful eating calls for a pause. Slow down, relish the moment, and let each morsel unfold its story on your palate.

3. **Listen to Your Body:** Tune into your body's cues. Are you truly hungry, or is it a response to emotions? Mindful eating encourages you to differentiate between physical hunger and emotional cravings.

4. **Gratitude for the Source:** Take a moment to acknowledge the journey your food has traveled – from seed to plate. Cultivate gratitude for the nourishment it provides and the hands involved in its cultivation.

Incorporating Mindfulness into Daily Life

Mindful eating transcends the confines of mealtime; it seamlessly integrates into your daily existence. Here are ways to infuse mindfulness beyond the dining table:

1. **Mindful Moments:** Embed mindful moments throughout your day. Whether it's sipping a cup of tea, walking in nature, or simply taking a few deep breaths, these pauses foster a sense of presence.

2. **Technology Detox:** Temporarily disconnect from the digital world during meals. Allow your focus to be solely on the culinary experience unfolding in front of you.

3. **Mindful Cooking:** Extend mindfulness to the kitchen. Engage with the ingredients, relish the

process of preparation, and infuse your creations with intention and joy.

4. **Cultivate Gratitude:** Take a moment each day to reflect on the abundance in your life. Express gratitude for the nourishment you receive, fostering a positive mindset.

Chapter 6 invites you to embrace the art of mindful eating, weaving a tapestry of health, gratitude, and presence into the fabric of your daily life. Through this practice, you'll discover that every meal is an opportunity for nourishment, connection, and a deeper understanding of yourself. May each bite be a celebration of life in its fullest expression.

CHAPTER SEVEN

Holistic Health and Wellness

Integrating Exercise with Diet

Step into the realm of holistic health and wellness with Chapter 7, where the synergy between exercise and diet unfolds as a cornerstone of your well-being. The marriage of these two elements forms a powerful alliance, laying the foundation for a life of vitality and balance.

Exercise is not merely a physical endeavor; it's a celebration of movement that echoes through the corridors of your entire being. In this chapter, discover how aligning your exercise routine with your dietary choices elevates the symphony of wellness. From invigorating workouts to the nourishment that fuels them, find the equilibrium that transforms your body into a temple of strength and resilience.

Stress Management Strategies

In the tapestry of holistic health, stress management emerges as a master weaver. Chapter 7 unveils an array of strategies to navigate the complexities of modern life without succumbing to chronic stress. As you delve into these practical tools, envision a life where stress is not an adversary but a catalyst for growth and resilience.

1. **Mindfulness Meditation:** Immerse yourself in the present moment through mindfulness meditation. This ancient practice becomes a beacon of tranquility in the storm of daily life.

2. **Breathwork Techniques:** Explore the profound impact of conscious breathing. Techniques such as

deep diaphragmatic breathing and alternate nostril breathing become your allies in restoring balance.

3. **Nature Immersion:** Reconnect with the healing power of nature. Whether it's a stroll in the park or a weekend getaway, nature has a unique ability to soothe the soul and ease the burdens of the mind.

4. **Holistic Therapies:** Delve into holistic therapies such as acupuncture, massage, or yoga. These time-honored practices become your companions on the journey to stress resilience.

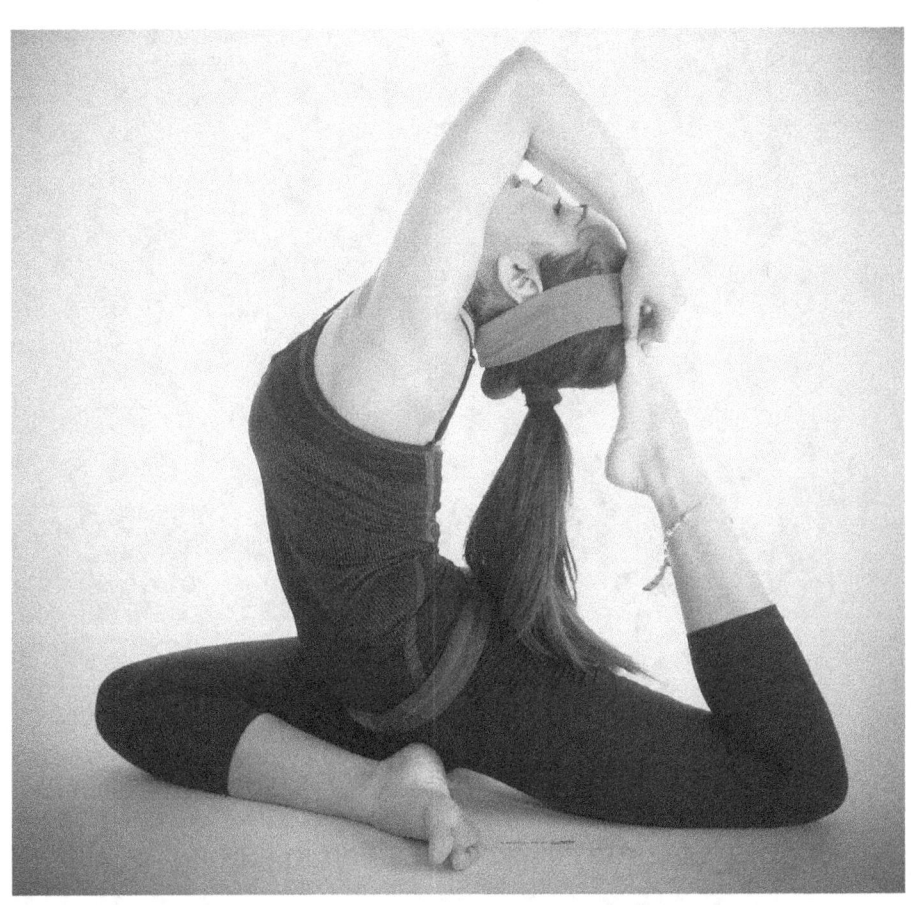

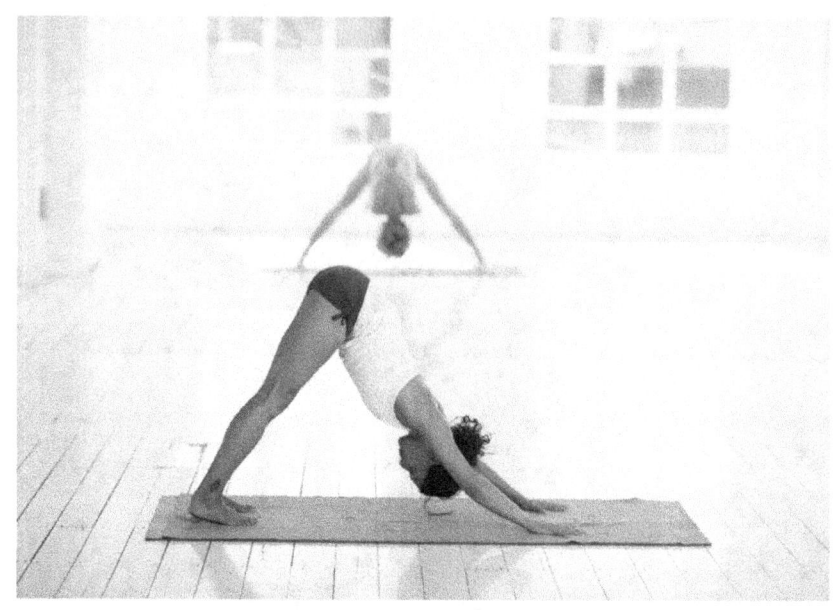

Sleep and its Role in Inflammation

Uncover the nocturnal wonders of Chapter 7 as we explore the profound role of sleep in taming the flames of inflammation. In the realm of holistic health, sleep is not a luxury but a vital elixir that rejuvenates mind, body, and spirit.

1. **Creating a Sleep Sanctuary:** Transform your bedroom into a haven of tranquility. From soothing

colors to comfortable bedding, design an environment that welcomes restful sleep.

2. **Establishing Sleep Routines:** Embrace the power of routines to signal your body that it's time to unwind. From consistent bedtimes to calming rituals, establish practices that invite a restful night.

3. **Screen Time Awareness:** Navigate the digital age with wisdom. Limit screen time before bedtime, allowing your mind to transition from the buzz of technology to the serenity of sleep.

4. **Nutrition for Sleep:** Discover the intricate dance between nutrition and sleep. Chapter 7 guides you through foods that promote restfulness, creating a culinary lullaby for your senses.

Chapter 7 invites you to weave the threads of exercise, stress management, and sleep into the intricate tapestry of your holistic well-being. As you embark on this transformative journey, envision a life where each choice is a brushstroke, painting a portrait of vitality, balance, and lasting wellness. May this chapter be your compass, guiding you toward a state of health that encompasses every facet of your being.

BONUS SECTION

Appetizers

1. Mango Avocado Salsa Cups

Description: Elevate your appetizer game with these refreshing mango avocado salsa cups. Bursting with vibrant colors and flavors, they're the perfect way to kick off any gathering.

Serving Size: 6 cups

Prep Time: 15 minutes

Ingredients:

- 2 ripe mangoes, diced

- 1 avocado, diced

- 1/2 red onion, finely chopped

- 1 jalapeño, seeded and minced

- Fresh cilantro, chopped

- Juice of 1 lime

- Salt and pepper to taste

- Tortilla cups for serving

Instructions:

1. In a bowl, combine diced mangoes, avocado, red onion, jalapeño, and cilantro.

2. Drizzle lime juice over the mixture and season with salt and pepper.

3. Gently toss until well combined.

4. Spoon the salsa into tortilla cups and serve chilled.

2. Caprese Bruschetta Bites

Description: Merge the classic flavors of Caprese with the beloved bruschetta in these delightful bites. A harmonious blend of tomatoes, mozzarella, and basil atop crusty bread makes for an appetizer that never disappoints.

Serving Size: 12 pieces

Prep Time: 15 minutes

Ingredients:

- 1 baguette, sliced

- 2 cups cherry tomatoes, halved

- 1 cup fresh mozzarella balls

- Fresh basil leaves

- Balsamic glaze for drizzling

- Olive oil for brushing

- Salt and pepper to taste

Instructions:

1. Preheat the oven to 375°F (190°C).

2. Arrange baguette slices on a baking sheet and brush with olive oil.

3. Bake for 8-10 minutes or until golden.

4. In a bowl, mix cherry tomatoes, mozzarella balls, and torn basil leaves.

5. Spoon the mixture onto the toasted baguette slices.

6. Drizzle with balsamic glaze and season with salt and pepper.

3. Spinach and Feta Stuffed Mushrooms

Description: These savory stuffed mushrooms are an irresistible combination of spinach and feta. A bite-sized delight that will vanish from the appetizer table in no time.

Serving Size: 24 mushrooms

Prep Time: 20 minutes

Cooking Time: 15 minutes

Ingredients:

- 24 large mushrooms, cleaned and stems removed

- 2 cups fresh spinach, chopped

- 1 cup feta cheese, crumbled

- 1/4 cup breadcrumbs

- 2 cloves garlic, minced

- 2 tablespoons olive oil

- Salt and pepper to taste

Instructions:

1. Preheat the oven to 375°F (190°C).

2. In a skillet, sauté spinach and garlic in olive oil until wilted.

3. In a bowl, combine spinach mixture, feta, breadcrumbs, salt, and pepper.

4. Stuff each mushroom cap with the mixture.

5. Place on a baking sheet and bake for 15 minutes or until mushrooms are tender.

4. Zucchini Ribbon Roll-Ups

Description: Embrace freshness with these zucchini ribbon roll-ups. Delicate zucchini strips are filled with herbed cream cheese, creating an appetizer that's light yet bursting with flavor.

Serving Size: 16 roll-ups

Prep Time: 15 minutes

Ingredients:

- 2 medium zucchinis, thinly sliced lengthwise

- 1 cup cream cheese, softened

- 1 tablespoon fresh dill, chopped

- 1 tablespoon chives, minced

- Zest of 1 lemon

- Salt and pepper to taste

Instructions:

1. In a bowl, mix softened cream cheese, dill, chives, lemon zest, salt, and pepper.

2. Lay out zucchini slices and spread a thin layer of the cream cheese mixture on each.

3. Roll up the zucchini slices and secure with toothpicks.

4. Chill in the refrigerator for at least 30 minutes before serving.

5. Crispy Baked Buffalo Cauliflower Bites

Description: Give a healthier twist to the classic buffalo wings with these crispy baked cauliflower bites. They're coated in a spicy buffalo sauce, creating a mouthwatering appetizer that's perfect for any gathering.

Serving Size: 4 servings

Prep Time: 15 minutes

Cooking Time: 25 minutes

Ingredients:

- 1 head cauliflower, cut into florets

- 1 cup flour

- 1 cup milk (or plant-based milk)

- 1 cup breadcrumbs

- 1/2 cup buffalo sauce

- 2 tablespoons melted butter (or vegan butter)

- Ranch or blue cheese dressing for dipping

Instructions:

1. Preheat the oven to 450°F (230°C).

2. In separate bowls, place flour, milk, and breadcrumbs.

3. Dip each cauliflower floret into the flour, then the milk, and finally coat with breadcrumbs.

4. Place coated florets on a baking sheet.

5. Bake for 20 minutes or until golden and crispy.

6. In a bowl, mix buffalo sauce and melted butter.

7. Toss baked cauliflower in the buffalo sauce mixture.

8. Serve with your choice of dressing for dipping.

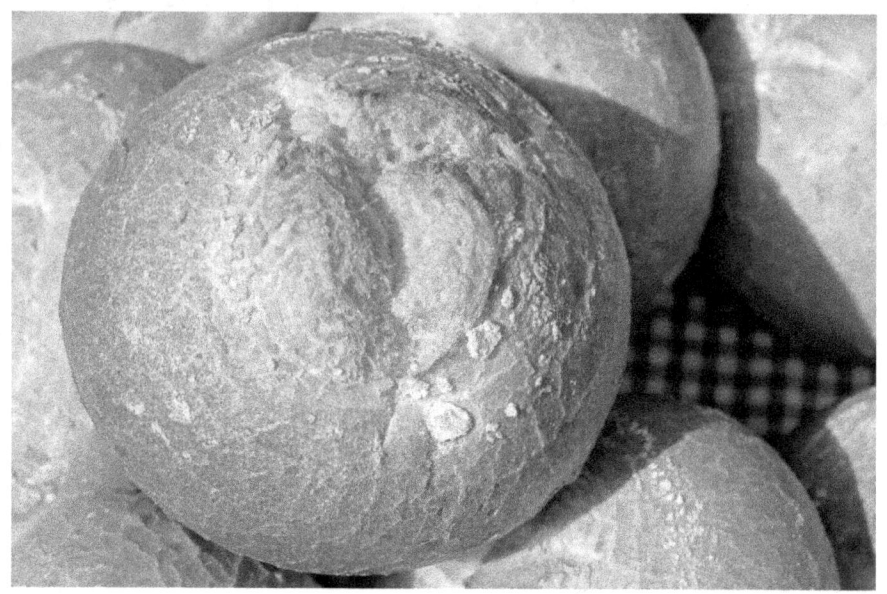

6. Smoked Salmon Cucumber Bites

Description: Experience the elegance of these smoked salmon cucumber bites. Creamy herbed cream cheese meets delicate smoked salmon, creating a bite-sized appetizer that's both sophisticated and delicious.

Serving Size: 12 pieces

Prep Time: 15 minutes

Ingredients:

- 1 English cucumber, sliced into rounds

- 4 oz smoked salmon

- 1/2 cup cream cheese, softened

- 1 tablespoon fresh dill, chopped

- 1 tablespoon capers

Instructions:

1. In a bowl, mix softened cream cheese and chopped dill.

2. Spread a small amount of the cream cheese mixture onto each cucumber round.

3. Top with a piece of smoked salmon and a few capers.

4. Arrange on a serving platter and refrigerate until ready to serve.

7. Stuffed Jalapeño Poppers

Description: Spice up your appetizer game with these stuffed jalapeño poppers. Creamy cheese, savory bacon, and a hint of spice make them a crowd-pleasing favorite.

Serving Size: 16 poppers

Prep Time: 20 minutes

Cooking Time: 15 minutes

Ingredients:

- 8 large jalapeños, halved and seeds removed

- 8 oz cream cheese, softened

- 1 cup shredded cheddar cheese

- 8 slices bacon, cooked and crumbled

- 1 teaspoon garlic powder

- Salt and pepper to taste

Instructions:

1. Preheat the oven to 375°F (190°C).

2. In a bowl, mix softened cream cheese, cheddar cheese, crumbled bacon, garlic powder, salt, and pepper.

3. Spoon the mixture into jalapeño halves.

4. Place on a baking sheet and bake for 15 minutes or until the cheese is melted and bubbly.

8. Mushroom and Goat Cheese Crostini

Description: Indulge in the earthy flavors of mushroom and goat cheese crostini. Sauteed mushrooms meet creamy goat cheese on a toasted baguette, creating a sophisticated appetizer that's simple yet elegant.

Serving Size: 12 pieces

Prep Time: 20 minutes

Cooking Time: 15 minutes

Ingredients:

- 1 baguette, sliced

- 2 cups mushrooms, sliced

- 4 oz goat cheese

- 2 tablespoons olive oil

- 2 cloves garlic, minced

- Fresh thyme leaves for garnish

- Salt and pepper to taste

Instructions:

1. Preheat the oven to 375°F (190°C).

2. Arrange baguette slices on a baking sheet and toast for 8-10 minutes or until golden.

3. In a skillet, sauté mushrooms and garlic in olive oil until softened.

4. Spread goat cheese on each baguette slice.

5. Top with sautéed mushrooms and garnish with fresh thyme leaves.

9. Sesame Ginger Edamame

Description: Introduce an Asian-inspired twist to your appetizer spread with these sesame ginger edamame pods. They're a flavorful and nutritious finger food that's both satisfying and delightful.

Serving Size: 4 servings

Prep Time: 10 minutes

Cooking Time: 5 minutes

Ingredients:

- 2 cups edamame pods (frozen and thawed)

- 2 tablespoons soy sauce

- 1 tablespoon sesame oil

- 1 tablespoon rice vinegar

- 1 teaspoon fresh ginger, grated

- 1 teaspoon sesame seeds

- Green onions for garnish

Instructions:

1. Boil edamame pods in salted water for 5 minutes, then drain.

2. In a bowl, whisk together soy sauce, sesame oil, rice vinegar, and grated ginger.

3. Toss the boiled edamame in the sauce mixture until well coated.

4. Sprinkle sesame seeds and garnish with chopped green onions.

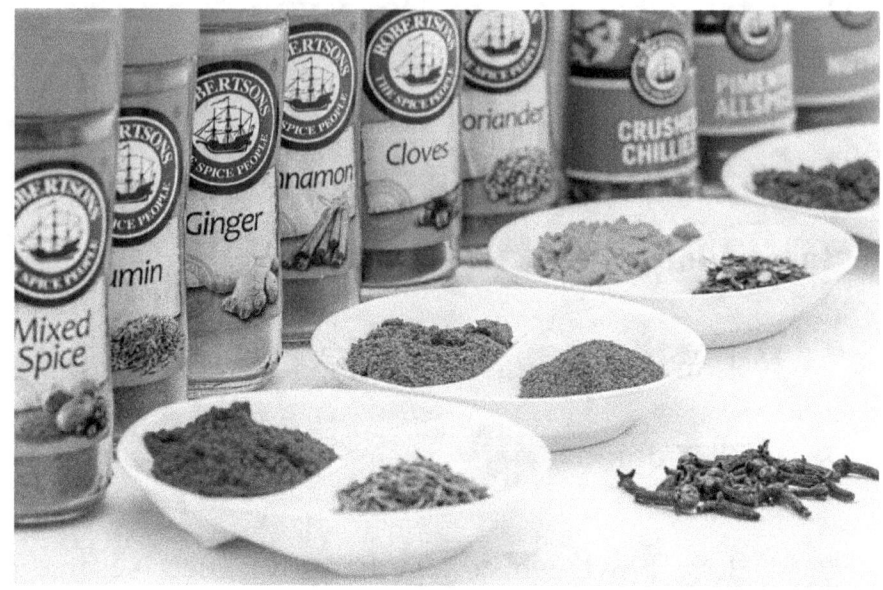

10. Artichoke and Spinach Dip Stuffed Breadsticks

Description: Transform the classic artichoke and spinach dip into a portable delight with these stuffed breadsticks. Each bite is a harmonious blend of cheesy goodness, making them a hit at any gathering.

Serving Size: 12 breadsticks

Prep Time: 25 minutes

Cooking Time: 15 minutes

Ingredients:

- 1 can (14 oz) artichoke hearts, drained and chopped

- 1 cup frozen chopped spinach, thawed and drained

- 1 cup shredded mozzarella cheese

- 1/2 cup grated Parmesan cheese

- 1/2 cup mayonnaise

- 1 teaspoon garlic powder

- Salt and pepper to taste

- 1 tube refrigerated breadsticks

Instructions:

1. Preheat the oven to 375°F (190°C).

2. In a bowl, mix chopped artichoke hearts, chopped spinach, mozzarella cheese, Parmesan cheese, mayonnaise, garlic powder, salt, and pepper.

3. Unroll the refrigerated breadsticks and separate them.

4. Spoon the artichoke and spinach mixture onto each breadstick and roll them up.

5. Place on a baking sheet and bake for 15 minutes or until golden.

Enjoy these appetizer recipes that promise to kickstart your gatherings with flavor and flair!

Soups and Salads

1. Roasted Tomato Basil Soup

Description: Experience the warmth and comfort of homemade Roasted Tomato Basil Soup. This classic recipe combines the sweetness of roasted tomatoes with the aromatic essence of fresh basil.

Serving Size: 4 servings

Prep Time: 15 minutes

Cooking Time: 45 minutes

Ingredients:

- 6 cups ripe tomatoes, halved

- 1/4 cup olive oil

- 1 onion, chopped

- 3 cloves garlic, minced

- 4 cups vegetable broth

- 1 cup fresh basil leaves

- Salt and pepper to taste

- Optional: Parmesan cheese for garnish

Instructions:

1. Preheat the oven to 400°F (200°C).

2. Toss halved tomatoes in olive oil, salt, and pepper. Roast for 30 minutes.

3. In a pot, sauté onion and garlic until softened.

4. Add roasted tomatoes and vegetable broth. Simmer for 15 minutes.

5. Blend the soup with fresh basil until smooth.

6. Season with salt and pepper. Garnish with Parmesan if desired.

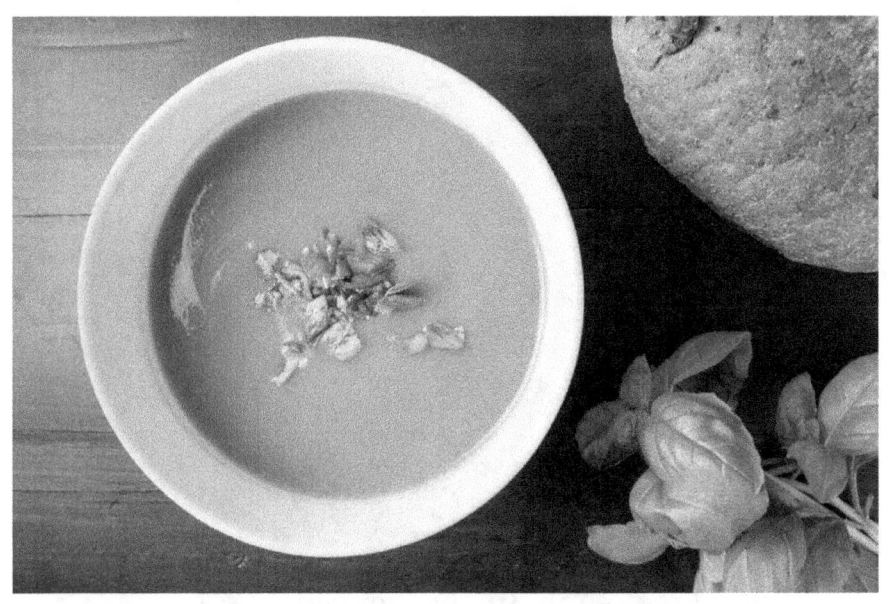

2. Quinoa and Chickpea Mediterranean Salad

Description: Transport your taste buds to the Mediterranean with this vibrant Quinoa and Chickpea Salad. Packed with protein, it's a refreshing and satisfying dish.

Serving Size: 6 servings

Prep Time: 20 minutes

Ingredients:

- 1 cup quinoa, cooked

- 1 can (15 oz) chickpeas, drained and rinsed

- 1 cucumber, diced

- 1 cup cherry tomatoes, halved

- 1/2 red onion, finely chopped

- 1/2 cup Kalamata olives, sliced

- 1/2 cup feta cheese, crumbled

- Fresh parsley, chopped

- Lemon vinaigrette dressing

Instructions:

1. In a large bowl, combine cooked quinoa, chickpeas, cucumber, cherry tomatoes, red onion, olives, and feta cheese.

2. Drizzle with lemon vinaigrette and toss to combine.

3. Garnish with fresh parsley before serving.

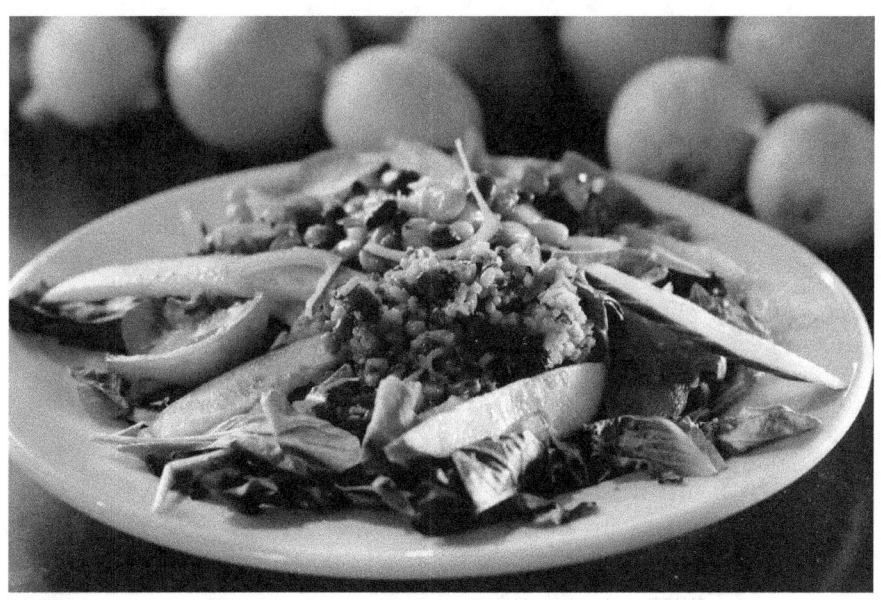

3. Butternut Squash and Apple Soup

Description: Celebrate the flavors of fall with this velvety Butternut Squash and Apple Soup. The sweetness of apples complements the earthy notes of butternut squash in this comforting bowl.

Serving Size: 6 servings

Prep Time: 20 minutes

Cooking Time: 40 minutes

Ingredients:

- 1 medium butternut squash, peeled and diced

- 2 apples, peeled and chopped

- 1 onion, chopped

- 2 carrots, chopped

- 4 cups vegetable broth

- 1 teaspoon curry powder

- 1/2 teaspoon nutmeg

- Salt and pepper to taste

- Coconut milk for garnish

Instructions:

1. In a pot, sauté onion until translucent. Add squash, apples, and carrots.

2. Pour in vegetable broth, curry powder, nutmeg, salt, and pepper. Simmer until vegetables are tender.

3. Blend the soup until smooth.

4. Serve hot, garnished with a swirl of coconut milk.

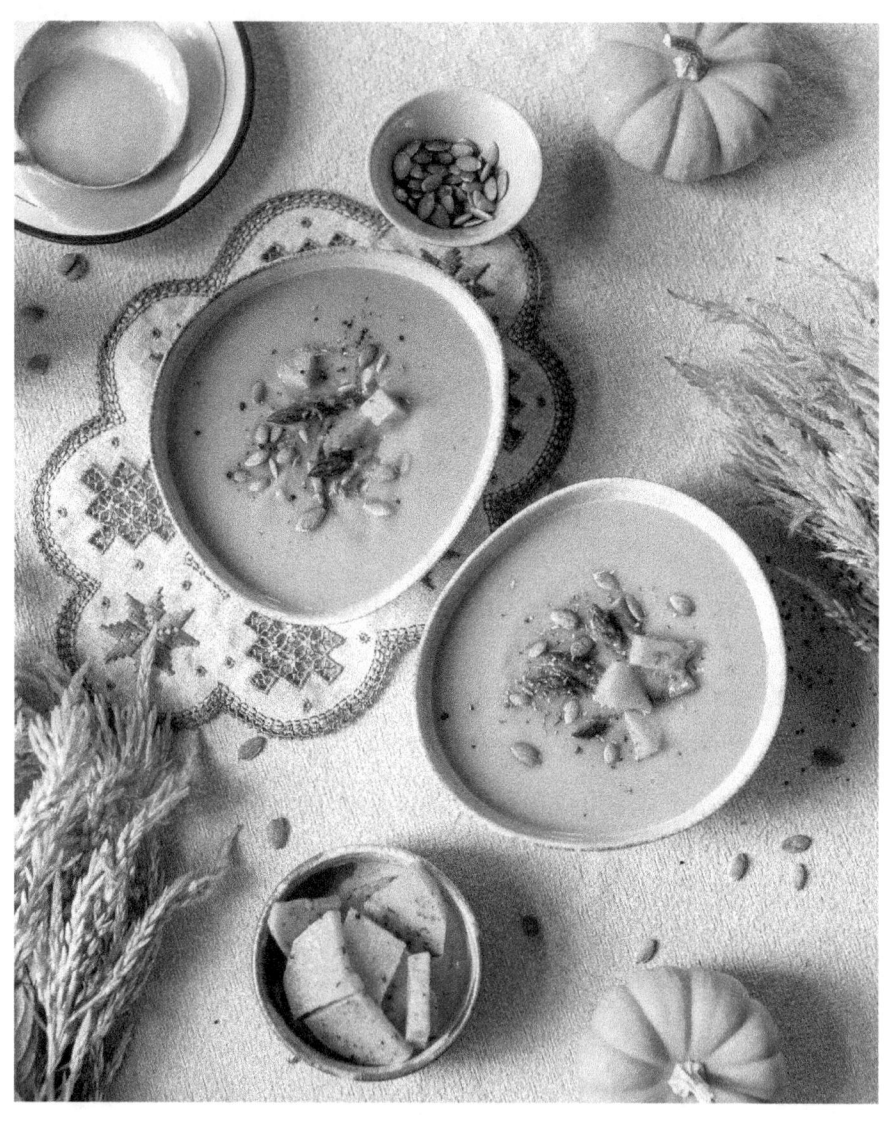

4. Kale and Quinoa Salad with Lemon Tahini Dressing

Description: Elevate your salad game with this nutrient-packed Kale and Quinoa Salad. The zesty Lemon Tahini Dressing adds a burst of flavor to this wholesome dish.

Serving Size: 4 servings

Prep Time: 15 minutes

Ingredients:

- 4 cups kale, destemmed and chopped

- 1 cup cooked quinoa

- 1 cup cherry tomatoes, halved

- 1 cucumber, sliced

- 1/2 red onion, thinly sliced

- 1/4 cup sunflower seeds

- Feta cheese (optional)

- Lemon Tahini Dressing

Instructions:

1. In a large bowl, massage kale with a bit of olive oil until softened.

2. Add quinoa, cherry tomatoes, cucumber, red onion, and sunflower seeds.

3. Drizzle with Lemon Tahini Dressing and toss to coat.

4. Top with feta cheese if desired before serving.

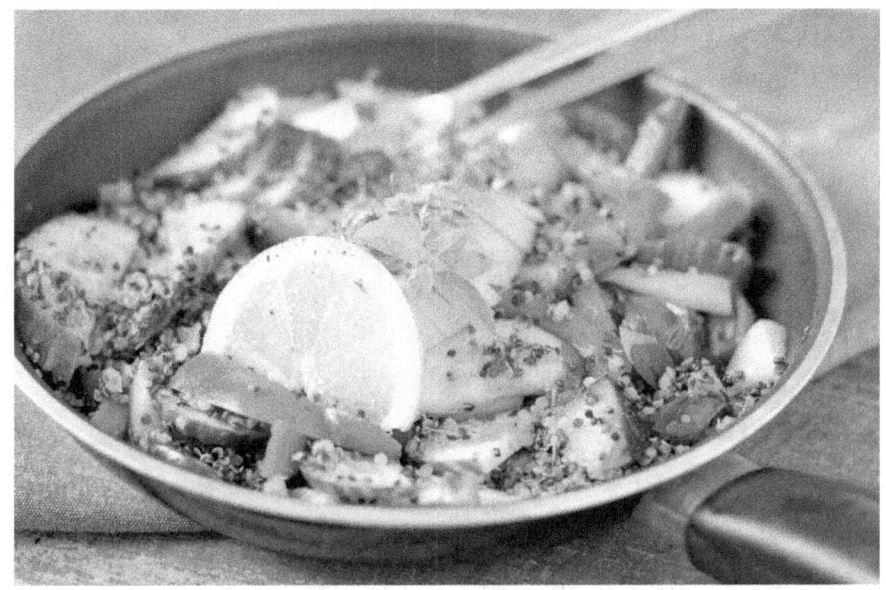

5. Chicken and Wild Rice Soup

Description: Embrace hearty goodness with Chicken and Wild Rice Soup. This soul-warming recipe blends tender chicken, nutty wild rice, and a medley of vegetables.

Serving Size: 6 servings

Prep Time: 15 minutes

Cooking Time: 45 minutes

Ingredients:

- 1 lb boneless, skinless chicken breasts, cubed

- 1 cup wild rice, uncooked

- 1 onion, chopped

- 3 carrots, sliced

- 3 celery stalks, chopped

- 4 cups chicken broth

- 1 teaspoon thyme

- 1/2 teaspoon garlic powder

- Salt and pepper to taste

Instructions:

1. In a pot, sauté chicken until browned. Remove and set aside.

2. In the same pot, sauté onion, carrots, and celery until softened.

3. Add chicken back to the pot, along with wild rice, chicken broth, thyme, garlic powder, salt, and pepper.

4. Simmer until rice is cooked and flavors meld.

6. Greek Orzo Salad

Description: Savor the freshness of the Mediterranean with this Greek Orzo Salad. Bursting with vibrant colors and bold flavors, it's a delightful addition to any meal.

Serving Size: 6 servings

Prep Time: 20 minutes

Cooking Time: 10 minutes

Ingredients:

- 1 cup orzo, cooked

- 1 cup cherry tomatoes, halved

- 1 cucumber, diced

- 1/2 red onion, finely chopped

- 1/2 cup Kalamata olives, sliced

- 1/2 cup feta cheese, crumbled

- Fresh parsley, chopped

- Greek vinaigrette dressing

Instructions:

1. In a large bowl, combine cooked orzo, cherry tomatoes, cucumber, red onion, olives, and feta cheese.

2. Drizzle with Greek vinaigrette and toss to combine.

3. Garnish with fresh parsley before serving.

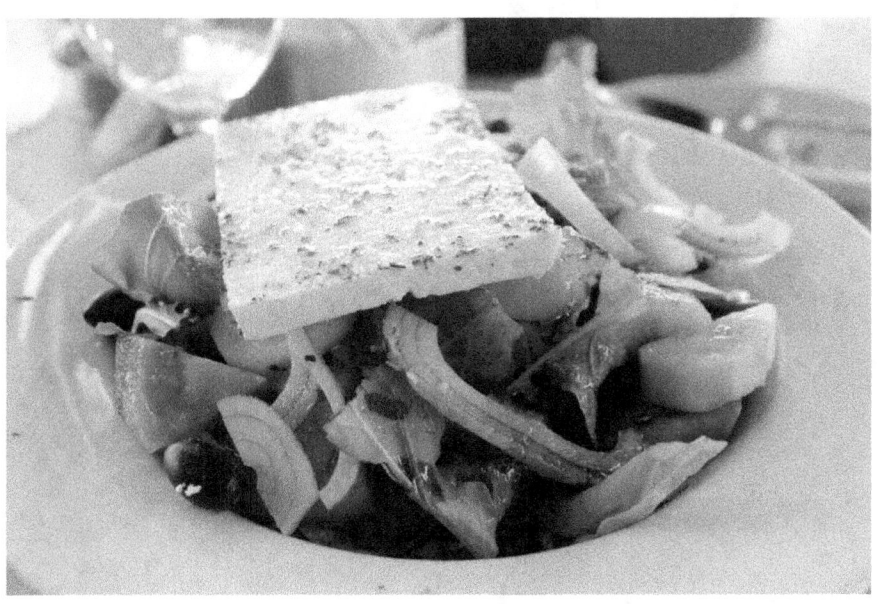

7. Lentil and Vegetable Soup

Description: Nourish your body with this hearty Lentil and Vegetable Soup. Packed with protein-rich lentils and an array of vegetables, it's a wholesome bowl of goodness.

Serving Size: 6 servings

Prep Time: 15 minutes

Cooking Time: 30 minutes

Ingredients:

- 1 cup dry green lentils, rinsed

- 1 onion, chopped

- 2 carrots, sliced

- 2 celery stalks, chopped

- 3 cloves garlic, minced

- 6 cups vegetable broth

- 1 can (14 oz) diced tomatoes

- 1 teaspoon cumin

- 1/2 teaspoon smoked paprika

- Salt and pepper to taste

Instructions:

1. In a pot, sauté onion, carrots, celery, and garlic until softened.

2. Add lentils, vegetable broth, diced tomatoes, cumin, smoked paprika, salt, and pepper.

3. Simmer until lentils are tender and flavors meld.

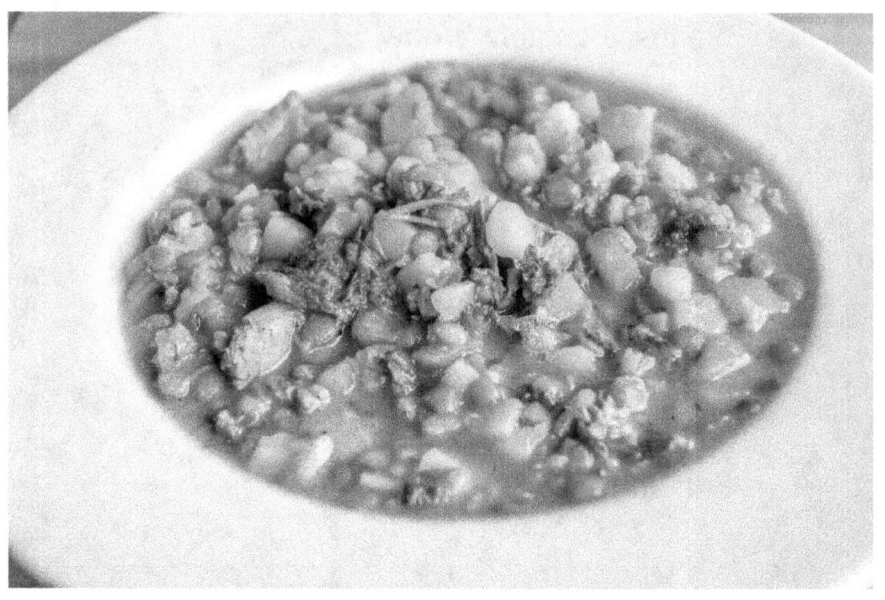

8. Caesar Salad with Grilled Chicken

Description: Indulge in the classic Caesar Salad with a protein boost from perfectly grilled chicken. Crisp romaine lettuce, parmesan, and homemade Caesar dressing create a timeless favorite.

Serving Size: 4 servings

Prep Time: 20 minutes

Cooking Time: 15 minutes

Ingredients:

- 2 boneless, skinless chicken breasts

- 1 head romaine lettuce, torn

- 1/2 cup croutons

- 1/4 cup parmesan cheese, shaved

- Caesar dressing (homemade or store-bought)

Instructions:

1. Grill chicken breasts until fully cooked, then slice.

2. In a large bowl, combine torn romaine lettuce, croutons, and shaved parmesan.

3. Top with grilled chicken slices.

4. Drizzle with Caesar dressing and toss to coat.

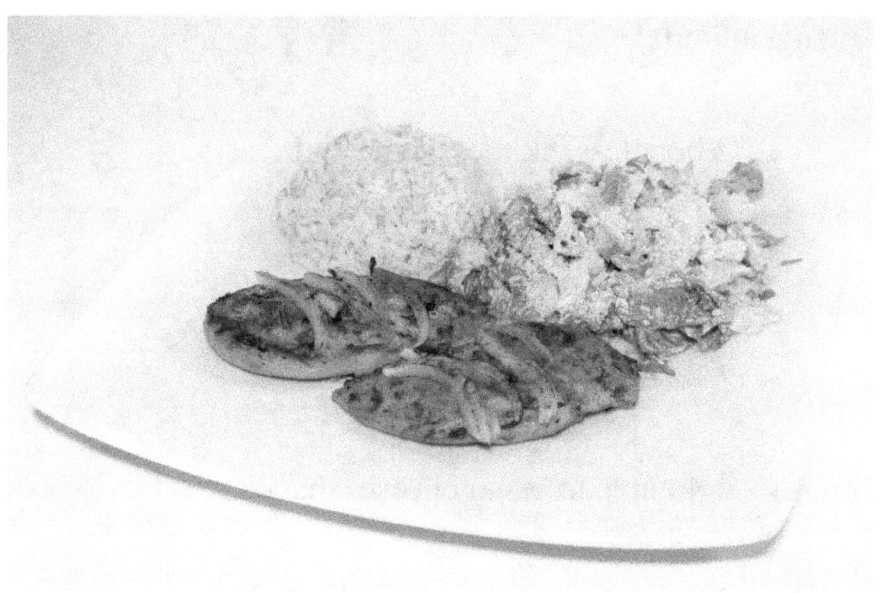

9. Creamy Broccoli Cheddar Soup

Description: Experience the cozy embrace of Creamy Broccoli Cheddar Soup. This velvety blend of broccoli and sharp cheddar creates a soup that's both comforting and decadent.

Serving Size: 4 servings

Prep Time: 15 minutes

Cooking Time: 25 minutes

Ingredients:

- 4 cups broccoli florets

- 1 onion, chopped

- 2 cloves garlic, minced

- 4 cups vegetable broth

- 1 cup sharp cheddar cheese, shredded

- 1/2 cup heavy cream

- 2 tablespoons flour

- Salt and pepper to taste

Instructions:

1. In a pot, sauté onion and garlic until softened.

2. Add broccoli and vegetable broth. Simmer until broccoli is tender.

3. In a separate bowl, whisk together flour and heavy cream.

4. Stir the cream mixture into the soup until thickened.

5. Add shredded cheddar, stirring until melted.

6. Season with salt and pepper.

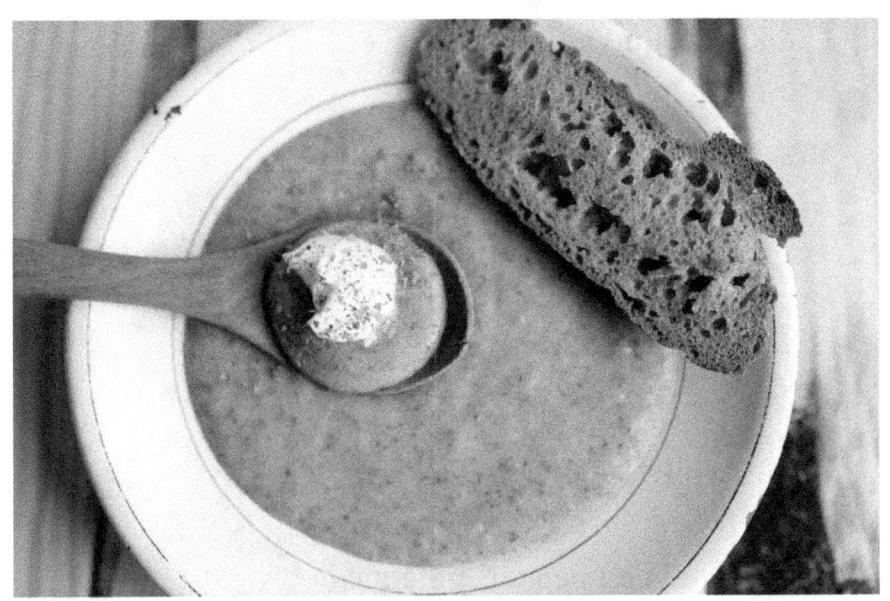

10. Asian-Inspired Noodle Salad

Description: Embark on a flavor journey with this Asian-Inspired Noodle Salad. Thin noodles mingle with vibrant vegetables and a zesty sesame ginger dressing for a delightful meal.

Serving Size: 4 servings

Prep Time: 15 minutes

Cooking Time: 10 minutes

Ingredients:

- 8 oz thin noodles (such as rice noodles or soba noodles)

- 1 cup snap peas, sliced

- 1 red bell pepper, julienned

- 1 carrot, shredded

- 1/4 cup green onions, chopped

- Sesame seeds for garnish

- Sesame ginger dressing

Instructions:

1. Cook noodles according to package instructions, then rinse under cold water.

2. In a large bowl, combine noodles, snap peas, red bell pepper, carrot, and green onions.

3. Drizzle with sesame ginger dressing and toss to coat.

4. Garnish with sesame seeds before serving.

Enjoy these soul-nourishing soups and salads that promise to bring a burst of flavor and wholesome goodness to your table!

Side Dishes

1. Garlic Parmesan Roasted Brussels Sprouts

Description: Elevate Brussels sprouts to a whole new level with this Garlic Parmesan Roasted Brussels Sprouts recipe. The combination of garlic and Parmesan adds a savory twist to these perfectly roasted sprouts.

Serving Size: 4 servings

Prep Time: 10 minutes

Cooking Time: 25 minutes

Ingredients:

- 1 lb Brussels sprouts, trimmed and halved

- 2 tablespoons olive oil

- 3 cloves garlic, minced

- 1/4 cup Parmesan cheese, grated

- Salt and pepper to taste

Instructions:

1. Preheat the oven to 400°F (200°C).

2. In a bowl, toss Brussels sprouts with olive oil, minced garlic, Parmesan cheese, salt, and pepper.

3. Spread them on a baking sheet in a single layer.

4. Roast for 20-25 minutes or until crispy and golden.

2. Crispy Parmesan Zucchini Fries

Description: Indulge in the crispy goodness of these Parmesan Zucchini Fries. Coated in Parmesan and baked to perfection, they make for a delightful and healthier alternative to traditional fries.

Serving Size: 4 servings

Prep Time: 15 minutes

Cooking Time: 20 minutes

Ingredients:

- 2 large zucchinis, cut into fries

- 1 cup Panko breadcrumbs

- 1/2 cup Parmesan cheese, grated

- 1 teaspoon Italian seasoning

- 2 eggs, beaten

- Salt and pepper to taste

Instructions:

1. Preheat the oven to 425°F (220°C).

2. In a bowl, combine Panko breadcrumbs, Parmesan, Italian seasoning, salt, and pepper.

3. Dip zucchini fries in beaten eggs, then coat with the breadcrumb mixture.

4. Place on a baking sheet and bake for 18-20 minutes or until golden and crispy.

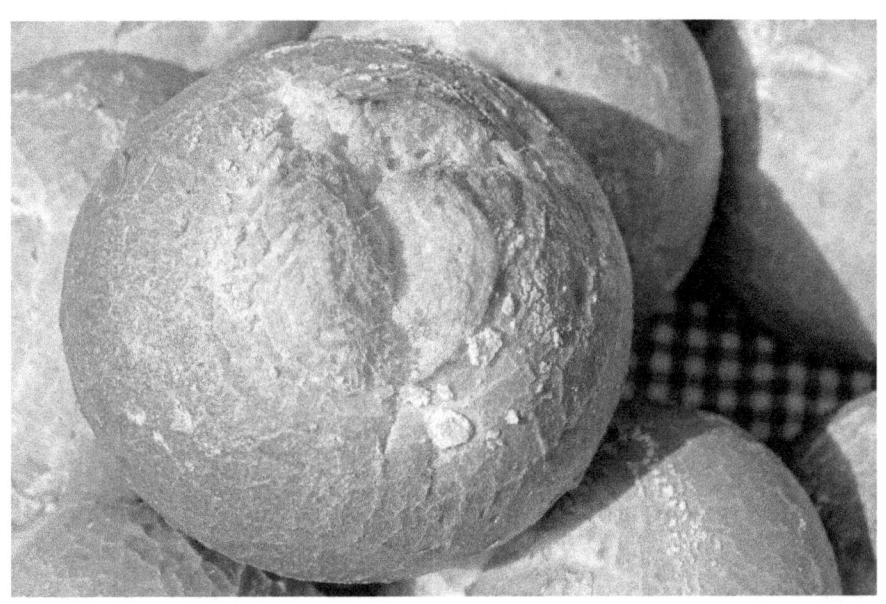

3. Mashed Sweet Potatoes with Maple Pecan Topping

Description: Turn ordinary sweet potatoes into a decadent delight with this Mashed Sweet Potatoes recipe. Topped with a luscious maple pecan topping, it's a side dish that feels like a dessert.

Serving Size: 6 servings

Prep Time: 15 minutes

Cooking Time: 20 minutes

Ingredients:

- 3 large sweet potatoes, peeled and cubed

- 1/4 cup butter

- 1/4 cup milk

- Salt and pepper to taste

- Topping: 1/4 cup chopped pecans, 2 tablespoons maple syrup

Instructions:

1. Boil sweet potatoes until tender. Drain and mash.

2. Mix in butter, milk, salt, and pepper.

3. In a separate pan, toast pecans until fragrant.

4. Drizzle maple syrup over the mashed sweet potatoes and sprinkle with toasted pecans.

4. Lemon Garlic Roasted Asparagus

Description: Brighten up your plate with the vibrant flavors of Lemon Garlic Roasted Asparagus. This simple yet elegant side dish brings out the best in asparagus with zesty lemon and savory garlic.

Serving Size: 4 servings

Prep Time: 10 minutes

Cooking Time: 15 minutes

Ingredients:

- 1 lb asparagus, trimmed

- 2 tablespoons olive oil

- 3 cloves garlic, minced

- Zest of 1 lemon

- Salt and pepper to taste

Instructions:

1. Preheat the oven to 400°F (200°C).

2. Toss asparagus with olive oil, minced garlic, lemon zest, salt, and pepper.

3. Spread on a baking sheet in a single layer.

4. Roast for 12-15 minutes or until tender-crisp.

5. Herbed Quinoa Pilaf

Description: Transform quinoa into a flavorful side dish with this Herbed Quinoa Pilaf. A medley of fresh herbs adds a burst of freshness to this wholesome and nutritious dish.

Serving Size: 4 servings

Prep Time: 10 minutes

Cooking Time: 20 minutes

Ingredients:

- 1 cup quinoa, rinsed

- 2 cups vegetable broth

- 2 tablespoons olive oil

- 1 onion, finely chopped

- 2 cloves garlic, minced

- 1/4 cup fresh parsley, chopped

- 1 tablespoon fresh dill, chopped

- Salt and pepper to taste

Instructions:

1. In a pot, sauté onion and garlic in olive oil until softened.

2. Add quinoa and toast for 2 minutes.

3. Pour in vegetable broth, bring to a boil, then reduce heat and simmer until quinoa is cooked.

4. Stir in fresh parsley and dill. Season with salt and pepper.

6. Honey Glazed Carrots with Thyme

Description: Elevate the humble carrot with this Honey Glazed Carrots with Thyme recipe. The natural sweetness of honey and the earthy aroma of thyme create a delightful side dish.

Serving Size: 4 servings

Prep Time: 10 minutes

Cooking Time: 15 minutes

Ingredients:

- 1 lb carrots, peeled and sliced

- 2 tablespoons butter

- 2 tablespoons honey

- Fresh thyme leaves

- Salt and pepper to taste

Instructions:

1. Boil or steam carrots until just tender. Drain.

2. In a pan, melt butter and honey together.

3. Add carrots and toss to coat in the honey-butter mixture.

4. Sprinkle with fresh thyme leaves, salt, and pepper.

7. Crispy Baked Parmesan Potato Wedges

Description: Satisfy your craving for crispy potatoes with these Baked Parmesan Potato Wedges. Oven-baked to perfection, they're a healthier alternative to traditional fries.

Serving Size: 4 servings

Prep Time: 15 minutes

Cooking Time: 30 minutes

Ingredients:

- 4 large potatoes, cut into wedges

- 2 tablespoons olive oil

- 1/2 cup Parmesan cheese, grated

- 1 teaspoon garlic powder

- 1 teaspoon paprika

- Salt and pepper to taste

Instructions:

1. Preheat the oven to 425°F (220°C).

2. Toss potato wedges with olive oil, Parmesan, garlic powder, paprika, salt, and pepper.

3. Spread on a baking sheet in a single layer.

4. Bake for 25-30 minutes or until golden and crispy.

8. Balsamic Glazed Roasted Vegetables

Description: Add a burst of flavor to your plate with Balsamic Glazed Roasted Vegetables. The rich balsamic glaze elevates the sweetness of the roasted vegetables for a mouthwatering side.

Serving Size: 4 servings

Prep Time: 15 minutes

Cooking Time: 30 minutes

Ingredients:

- 2 cups mixed vegetables (e.g., bell peppers, cherry tomatoes, zucchini)

- 2 tablespoons olive oil

- 2 tablespoons balsamic glaze

- Salt and pepper to taste

Instructions:

1. Preheat the oven to 400°F (200°C).

2. Toss mixed vegetables with olive oil, salt, and pepper.

3. Roast for 20-25 minutes or until vegetables are tender.

4. Drizzle with balsamic glaze before serving.

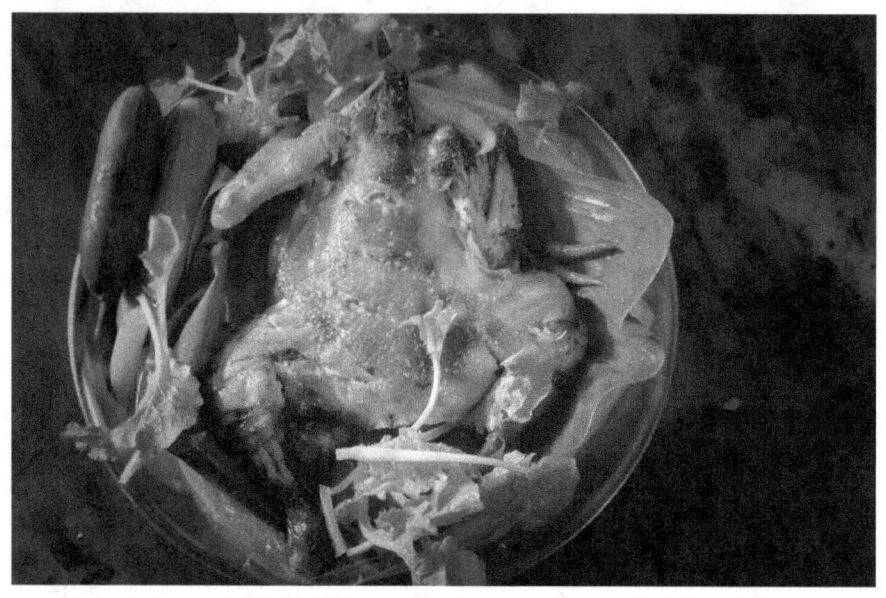

9. Creamy Garlic Parmesan Risotto

Description: Indulge in the creamy goodness of Garlic Parmesan Risotto. This classic Italian dish combines Arborio rice with garlic and Parmesan for a rich and satisfying side.

Serving Size: 4 servings

Prep Time: 10 minutes

Cooking Time: 25 minutes

Ingredients:

- 1 cup Arborio rice

- 4 cups chicken or vegetable broth, warmed

- 2 tablespoons butter

- 2 cloves garlic, minced

- 1/2 cup Parmesan cheese, grated

- Salt and pepper to taste

- Fresh parsley for garnish

Instructions:

1. In a pan, sauté garlic in butter until fragrant.

2. Add Arborio rice and cook for 2 minutes.

3. Gradually add warm broth, one ladle at a time, stirring until absorbed.

4. Continue until the rice is creamy and cooked al dente.

5. Stir in Parmesan cheese, salt, and pepper. Garnish with fresh parsley.

10. Grilled Corn with Chili Lime Butter

Description: Celebrate the flavors of summer with Grilled Corn with Chili Lime Butter. This side dish brings the sweetness of grilled corn together with zesty chili lime butter for a delightful treat.

Serving Size: 4 servings

Prep Time: 10 minutes

Cooking Time: 10 minutes

Ingredients:

- 4 ears of corn, husked

- 4 tablespoons unsalted butter, softened

- Zest and juice of 1 lime

- 1 teaspoon chili powder

- Salt to taste

Instructions:

1. Preheat the grill to medium-high heat.

2. Grill corn until slightly charred, turning occasionally.

3. In a bowl, mix softened butter, lime zest, lime juice, chili powder, and salt.

4. Spread the chili lime butter over the grilled corn before serving.

Enjoy these side dishes that promise to complement your main course with a burst of flavor and variety!

Desserts

1. Dark Chocolate Avocado Mousse

Description: Indulge in the richness of this Dark Chocolate Avocado Mousse. Creamy avocados combine with dark chocolate for a decadent and healthier dessert that's both satisfying and guilt-free.

Serving Size: 4 servings

Prep Time: 15 minutes

Ingredients:

- 2 ripe avocados

- 1/2 cup dark chocolate, melted

- 1/4 cup cocoa powder

- 1/4 cup maple syrup or honey

- 1 teaspoon vanilla extract

- Pinch of salt

- Fresh berries for garnish

Instructions:

1. In a blender or food processor, combine avocados, melted dark chocolate, cocoa powder, maple syrup, vanilla extract, and a pinch of salt.

2. Blend until smooth and creamy.

3. Chill in the refrigerator for at least 1 hour.

4. Serve topped with fresh berries.

2. Raspberry Almond Chia Pudding

Description: Savor the delightful combination of tart raspberries and crunchy almonds in this Raspberry Almond Chia Pudding. This nutritious dessert is a perfect balance of sweetness and texture.

Serving Size: 4 servings

Prep Time: 10 minutes

Ingredients:

- 1/2 cup chia seeds

- 2 cups almond milk

- 1 teaspoon vanilla extract

- 1 tablespoon maple syrup or agave

- 1 cup fresh raspberries

- 1/4 cup sliced almonds

Instructions:

1. In a bowl, mix chia seeds, almond milk, vanilla extract, and maple syrup.

2. Stir well and let it sit for 10 minutes, stirring occasionally.

3. Layer the chia pudding with fresh raspberries in serving glasses.

4. Top with sliced almonds before serving.

3. Coconut Mango Sticky Rice

Description: Transport your taste buds to tropical bliss with Coconut Mango Sticky Rice. This Thai-inspired dessert combines sweet mango with coconut-infused sticky rice for a heavenly treat.

Serving Size: 4 servings

Prep Time: 20 minutes

Cooking Time: 20 minutes

Ingredients:

- 1 cup glutinous rice, soaked for 1 hour

- 1 can (14 oz) coconut milk

- 1/2 cup sugar

- 1/2 teaspoon salt

- 2 ripe mangoes, sliced

- Sesame seeds for garnish

Instructions:

1. Rinse soaked glutinous rice and steam for 20 minutes or until tender.

2. In a saucepan, heat coconut milk, sugar, and salt until dissolved.

3. Pour the coconut mixture over the cooked rice and let it soak for 15 minutes.

4. Serve sticky rice topped with sliced mangoes and a sprinkle of sesame seeds.

4. Pistachio Cardamom Energy Bites

Description: Fuel your sweet cravings with these Pistachio Cardamom Energy Bites. Packed with nutrient-dense ingredients, these bites offer a delightful blend of pistachios and aromatic cardamom.

Serving Size: 12 bites

Prep Time: 15 minutes

Ingredients:

- 1 cup shelled pistachios

- 1 cup dates, pitted

- 1/2 cup rolled oats

- 1 teaspoon ground cardamom

- 1/4 cup honey or agave nectar

- Pinch of salt

- Shredded coconut for coating

Instructions:

1. In a food processor, blend pistachios, dates, rolled oats, cardamom, honey, and a pinch of salt until well combined.

2. Roll the mixture into bite-sized balls.

3. Coat each energy bite with shredded coconut.

4. Chill in the refrigerator for at least 30 minutes before serving.

5. Banana Walnut Bread Pudding

Description: Experience the warmth of comfort with this Banana Walnut Bread Pudding. Ripe bananas and toasted walnuts come together in this cozy and irresistible dessert.

Serving Size: 6 servings

Prep Time: 15 minutes

Cooking Time: 45 minutes

Ingredients:

- 4 cups stale bread, cubed

- 2 ripe bananas, mashed

- 1/2 cup chopped walnuts, toasted

- 2 cups milk

- 3/4 cup sugar

- 3 eggs

- 1 teaspoon vanilla extract

- Pinch of cinnamon

- Maple syrup for drizzling

Instructions:

1. Preheat the oven to 350°F (175°C).

2. In a bowl, combine bread cubes, mashed bananas, and toasted walnuts.

3. In another bowl, whisk together milk, sugar, eggs, vanilla extract, and cinnamon.

4. Pour the milk mixture over the bread mixture, ensuring everything is coated.

5. Let it sit for 15 minutes, then transfer to a baking dish.

6. Bake for 45 minutes or until golden and set.

7. Drizzle with maple syrup before serving.

6. Chia Seed Chocolate Pudding

Description: Delight in the velvety goodness of Chia Seed Chocolate Pudding. This no-bake dessert is a healthy twist on chocolate pudding, featuring the nutritious goodness of chia seeds.

Serving Size: 4 servings

Prep Time: 10 minutes

Chilling Time: 4 hours or overnight

Ingredients:

- 1/2 cup chia seeds

- 2 cups almond milk

- 1/4 cup cocoa powder

- 1/4 cup maple syrup or honey

- 1 teaspoon vanilla extract

- Fresh berries for topping

Instructions:

1. In a bowl, whisk together chia seeds, almond milk, cocoa powder, maple syrup, and vanilla extract.

2. Let it sit for 10 minutes, stirring occasionally.

3. Cover and refrigerate for at least 4 hours or overnight.

4. Serve topped with fresh berries.

7. Apple Cinnamon Oatmeal Cookies

Description: Satisfy your sweet tooth with these Apple Cinnamon Oatmeal Cookies. Bursting with the flavors of apple and warm cinnamon, these cookies are a delightful treat any time of day.

Serving Size: 18 cookies

Prep Time: 15 minutes

Cooking Time: 12 minutes

Ingredients:

- 1 cup rolled oats

- 3/4 cup whole wheat flour

- 1/2 teaspoon baking soda

- 1/2 teaspoon ground cinnamon

- 1/4 teaspoon salt

- 1/4 cup coconut oil, melted

- 1/4 cup maple syrup or honey

- 1 egg

- 1 teaspoon vanilla extract

- 1 apple, grated

- 1/2 cup chopped walnuts (optional)

Instructions:

1. Preheat the oven to 350°F (175°C).

2. In a bowl, combine rolled oats, whole wheat flour, baking soda, cinnamon, and salt.

3. In another bowl, whisk together melted coconut oil, maple syrup, egg, and vanilla extract.

4. Mix wet ingredients into the dry ingredients.

5. Fold in grated apple and chopped walnuts (if using).

6. Drop spoonfuls of dough onto a baking sheet.

7. Bake for 12 minutes or until golden around the edges.

8. Strawberry Cheesecake Parfait

Description: Indulge in the elegance of this Strawberry Cheesecake Parfait. Layers of creamy cheesecake filling and sweet strawberries create a delightful dessert that's both visually appealing and delicious.

Serving Size: 4 servings

Prep Time: 20 minutes

Ingredients:

- 1 cup cream cheese, softened

- 1/2 cup Greek yogurt

- 1/4 cup powdered sugar

- 1 teaspoon vanilla extract

- 2 cups fresh strawberries, sliced

- Graham cracker crumbs for layering

Instructions:

1. In a bowl, beat together cream cheese, Greek yogurt, powdered sugar, and vanilla extract until smooth.

2. In serving glasses, layer the cheesecake mixture with sliced strawberries and graham cracker crumbs.

3. Repeat the layers until the glasses are filled.

4. Refrigerate for at least 1 hour before serving.

9. Almond Flour Chocolate Chip Cookies

Description: Experience the perfect balance of chewiness and chocolatey goodness with these Almond Flour Chocolate Chip Cookies. Made with almond flour, they're a gluten-free delight.

Serving Size: 18 cookies

Prep Time: 15 minutes

Cooking Time: 10 minutes

Ingredients:

- 2 cups almond flour

- 1/2 teaspoon baking soda

- 1/4 teaspoon salt

- 1/4 cup coconut oil, melted

- 1/4 cup maple syrup or honey

- 1 egg

- 1 teaspoon vanilla extract

- 1/2 cup dark chocolate chips

Instructions:

1. Preheat the oven to 350°F (175°C).

2. In a bowl, combine almond flour, baking soda, and salt.

3. In another bowl, whisk together melted coconut oil, maple syrup, egg, and vanilla extract.

4. Mix wet ingredients into the dry ingredients.

5. Fold in dark chocolate chips.

6. Drop spoonfuls of dough onto a baking sheet.

7. Bake for 10 minutes or until golden.

10. Pumpkin Spice Energy Bites

Description: Embrace the cozy flavors of fall with these Pumpkin Spice Energy Bites. Packed with pumpkin, warm spices, and rolled oats, they're a nutritious and flavorful treat.

Serving Size: 12 bites

Prep Time: 15 minutes

Ingredients:

- 1 cup rolled oats

- 1/2 cup pumpkin puree

- 1/4 cup almond butter

- 1/4 cup honey

- 1 teaspoon pumpkin spice

- 1/2 cup shredded coconut for rolling

Instructions:

1. In a bowl, mix together rolled oats, pumpkin puree, almond butter, honey, and pumpkin spice.

2. Roll the mixture into bite-sized balls.

3. Coat each energy bite with shredded coconut.

4. Chill in the refrigerator for at least 30 minutes before serving.

Enjoy these delectable desserts that promise to satisfy your sweet cravings with wholesome ingredients and delightful flavors!

Drinks

1. Matcha Green Tea Latte

Description: Elevate your tea experience with the vibrant Matcha Green Tea Latte. Rich in antioxidants, this frothy and comforting beverage is a perfect balance of earthy matcha and velvety milk.

Serving Size: 2 servings

Prep Time: 5 minutes

Ingredients:

- 2 teaspoons matcha powder

- 2 cups milk (dairy or plant-based)

- 2 tablespoons honey or sweetener of choice

Instructions:

1. In a bowl, whisk matcha powder with a small amount of hot water until smooth.

2. Heat milk in a saucepan until steaming but not boiling.

3. Pour the hot milk over the matcha mixture.

4. Add honey or sweetener and whisk until frothy.

5. Pour into mugs and enjoy.

2. Berry Citrus Smoothie

Description: Revitalize your day with the refreshing Berry Citrus Smoothie. Packed with vitamins and antioxidants, this vibrant blend of berries and citrus is a delightful burst of flavor.

Serving Size: 2 servings

Prep Time: 5 minutes

Ingredients:

- 1 cup mixed berries (strawberries, blueberries, raspberries)

- 1 orange, peeled and segmented

- 1 banana

- 1 cup yogurt (dairy or plant-based)

- 1 tablespoon honey or agave nectar

- Ice cubes (optional)

Instructions:

1. In a blender, combine mixed berries, orange segments, banana, yogurt, and honey.

2. Blend until smooth and creamy.

3. Add ice cubes if desired and blend again.

4. Pour into glasses and enjoy the fruity goodness.

3. Turmeric Golden Milk

Description: Embrace the warmth and wellness of Turmeric Golden Milk. This soothing and anti-inflammatory beverage combines turmeric, ginger, and spices for a comforting drink.

Serving Size: 2 servings

Prep Time: 5 minutes

Cooking Time: 10 minutes

Ingredients:

- 2 cups milk (dairy or plant-based)

- 1 teaspoon ground turmeric

- 1/2 teaspoon ground ginger

- 1/4 teaspoon ground cinnamon

- Pinch of black pepper

- 1 tablespoon honey or maple syrup

Instructions:

1. In a small saucepan, heat milk over medium heat.

2. Add turmeric, ginger, cinnamon, and black pepper.

3. Whisk continuously until heated but not boiling.

4. Remove from heat, add honey or maple syrup, and whisk again.

5. Pour into mugs, straining if needed, and savor the golden warmth.

4. Cucumber Mint Lemonade

Description: Quench your thirst with the refreshing Cucumber Mint Lemonade. This invigorating drink combines the crispness of cucumber, the brightness of lemon, and the coolness of mint.

Serving Size: 4 servings

Prep Time: 10 minutes

Ingredients:

- 2 cucumbers, peeled and sliced

- 1/2 cup fresh mint leaves

- 1 cup freshly squeezed lemon juice

- 1/2 cup honey or agave nectar

- 4 cups water

- Ice cubes

Instructions:

1. In a blender, combine cucumber slices, mint leaves, lemon juice, and honey.

2. Blend until smooth.

3. Strain the mixture into a pitcher to remove pulp.

4. Add water and stir well.

5. Serve over ice and garnish with mint leaves.

5. Iced Rooibos Hibiscus Tea

Description: Cool down with the vibrant Iced Rooibos Hibiscus Tea. This caffeine-free and fruity blend of rooibos and hibiscus is a perfect sip for a sunny day.

Serving Size: 2 servings

Prep Time: 5 minutes

Ingredients:

- 2 rooibos tea bags

- 2 hibiscus tea bags

- 4 cups boiling water

- 2 tablespoons honey or agave nectar

- Lemon slices and mint for garnish

- Ice cubes

Instructions:

1. Steep rooibos and hibiscus tea bags in boiling water for 5-7 minutes.

2. Remove tea bags and stir in honey or agave nectar.

3. Let the tea cool, then refrigerate until cold.

4. Fill glasses with ice cubes and pour the chilled tea over.

5. Garnish with lemon slices and mint.

6. Pineapple Ginger Sparkler

Description: Sparkle up your day with the Pineapple Ginger Sparkler. This effervescent and tropical drink combines the zing of ginger with the sweetness of pineapple for a bubbly treat.

Serving Size: 2 servings

Prep Time: 10 minutes

Ingredients:

- 1 cup fresh pineapple chunks

- 1-inch piece of ginger, peeled and sliced

- 2 cups sparkling water

- 1 tablespoon honey or agave nectar

- Ice cubes

- Pineapple wedges for garnish

Instructions:

1. In a blender, blend pineapple chunks and sliced ginger until smooth.

2. Strain the mixture into a pitcher.

3. Add sparkling water and honey, stirring until well combined.

4. Fill glasses with ice cubes and pour the pineapple ginger mixture over.

5. Garnish with pineapple wedges and enjoy the fizz.

7. Mango Lassi

Description: Transport yourself to the tropics with the luscious Mango Lassi. This traditional Indian drink combines ripe mangoes, yogurt, and a touch of cardamom for a creamy delight.

Serving Size: 2 servings

Prep Time: 5 minutes

Ingredients:

- 2 ripe mangoes, peeled and diced

- 1 cup yogurt (dairy or plant-based)

- 1/2 cup milk (dairy or plant-based)

- 2 tablespoons honey or agave nectar

- 1/4 teaspoon ground cardamom

- Ice cubes

Instructions:

1. In a blender, blend mangoes, yogurt, milk, honey, and cardamom until smooth.

2. Add ice cubes and blend again until creamy.

3. Pour into glasses and savor the tropical goodness.

8. Cold Brew Coffee with Vanilla Almond Milk

Description: Experience the smoothness of Cold Brew Coffee with Vanilla Almond Milk. This chilled coffee delight is infused with the nutty richness of almond milk and a hint of vanilla.

Serving Size: 2 servings

Prep Time: 5 minutes

Brewing Time: 12-24 hours

Ingredients:

- 1/2 cup coarsely ground coffee

- 2 cups cold water

- 1 cup vanilla almond milk

- 1-2 tablespoons maple syrup or sweetener of choice

- Ice cubes

Instructions:

1. Combine coarsely ground coffee and cold water in a jar.

2. Stir well, cover, and refrigerate for 12-24 hours.

3. Strain the coffee concentrate into a pitcher.

4. Mix in vanilla almond milk and sweetener.

5. Serve over ice and enjoy the velvety richness.

9. Watermelon Basil Infused Water

Description: Stay hydrated with the revitalizing Watermelon Basil Infused Water. This naturally flavored water combines juicy watermelon and fragrant basil for a refreshing twist.

Serving Size: 4 servings

Prep Time: 5 minutes

Ingredients:

- 2 cups watermelon cubes

- 1/4 cup fresh basil leaves

- 4 cups cold water

- Ice cubes

Instructions:

1. In a pitcher, combine watermelon cubes and fresh basil leaves.

2. Add cold water and stir gently.

3. Refrigerate for at least 1 hour to let the flavors infuse.

4. Serve over ice and enjoy the subtly sweet hydration.

10. Chamomile Lavender Sleepy Tea

Description: Unwind with the soothing Chamomile Lavender Sleepy Tea. This calming blend of chamomile and lavender is perfect for a relaxing evening ritual before bedtime.

Serving Size: 2 servings

Prep Time: 5 minutes

Ingredients:

- 2 chamomile tea bags

- 1 teaspoon dried lavender

- 2 cups boiling water

- 1-2 tablespoons honey or agave nectar (optional)

Instructions:

1. Steep chamomile tea bags and dried lavender in boiling water for 5 minutes.

2. Remove tea bags and strain the tea to remove lavender.

3. Sweeten with honey or agave nectar if desired.

4. Sip slowly and embrace the tranquility.

Enjoy these diverse and flavorful drink recipes that cater to various preferences and occasions!

CONCLUSION

As we wrap up this journey through the pages of the **"Anti-Inflammatory Diet Cookbook,"** it is my sincere hope that the vibrant recipes and insightful guidance have not only nourished your body but ignited a transformation in your approach to holistic well-being.

In the culinary landscape we've traversed, each dish is not merely a combination of ingredients; it is a symphony of flavors meticulously orchestrated to harmonize with the intricate rhythms of your health. From the science of inflammation to the practicalities of meal planning, we've endeavored to simplify the path to wellness.

This cookbook goes beyond the kitchen; it is an invitation to a lifestyle—a lifestyle centered on mindful nourishment, where every bite is a step towards embracing vitality. The connection between what we consume and how we feel is profound, and with this awareness, you hold the reins to your well-being.

As you embark on your culinary adventures, remember that wellness is a continuous journey, not a destination. It is the sum of daily choices, the mindful selection of ingredients, and the joy found in savoring each meal. This book is not just a collection of recipes; it is a companion on your path to a more vibrant, healthier you.

May the flavors linger on your palate, reminding you of the delightful journey you've undertaken towards simplified wellness. Let this book be your guide, empowering you to craft not just meals but a lifestyle steeped in nourishment, balance, and the pure joy of living well.

Here's to your health, happiness, and the delicious journey ahead!